Dorot
It m
make this row
row contact with
you!
Uncle Hank
Jan. / 22

CREEKS
AND
CRISES

*T*HEN AND *N*OW

HANK NEUFELD

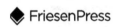 FriesenPress

One Printers Way
Altona, MB R0G 0B0
Canada

www.friesenpress.com

ISBN
978-1-03-912406-6 (Hardcover)
978-1-03-912405-9 (Paperback)
978-1-03-912407-3 (eBook)

1. BIOGRAPHY & AUTOBIOGRAPHY, PERSONAL MEMOIRS

Distributed to the trade by The Ingram Book Company

Dedication

A few years ago, my wife Betty and I spent an evening with two adult nieces whom we had not seen for decades. After a few delightful hours, they expressed their regret for not having known us sooner and better. I jotted down a few notes the next day and this memoir was conceived. It is sincerely dedicated to our fifty-six nephews and nieces, and our two grandchildren. We wish them all a life of excitement, achievement, and goodwill.

TABLE OF CONTENTS

Age Twenty-three to Twenty-nine

PART II

PART I

Preface

My ancestral roots lie in the Netherlands. There, Menno Simons (1496–1561), a friend to Martin Luther, led his followers away from the established church and founded a Protestant group that took his name: Mennonites.

What distinguished Mennonites from other Protestants was their commitment to freedom of religion (including rejection of child baptism) and pacifism (refusal to participate in direct war efforts). For hundreds of years, Mennonites stood firm in choosing their own conditions for citizenship, even when this stance ultimately drove them from Holland to Switzerland, Germany, Poland, Canada, Prussia, South America, Russia – and almost any country that promised freedom of religion and exemption from military service.

Introduction

I began this memoir by writing my autobiography. I had far too much material and, at eighty, too little time. A segment of my life, a memoir, was called for. But what to drop? I chose to include the early part of my life and the last, my retirement. My working life deserves another memoir.

Most memoir writers research dates, name relevant people, and draw up a sequential order of main events. A memoir such as mine also tries to be relatively accurate with dates, events and identities, but tries to do more. Memoirs can achieve a higher interest level by depicting many diverse scenes by telling narratives, or little stories that include well-informed estimates of the details between events. These vignettes continue until they uncover the bigger story, in my case two specific parts of my life. I have mostly used real names, and pseudonyms on occasion. Other people critical to my life may be recognized by their actions and personal peculiarities.

This memoir recalls the core or kernel of "what happened" and the distinctive tone or timbre of what was said. Nobody can remember the exact words of conversations held long ago, but by summoning up the essence of events, I broaden the story so that it is based on the atmosphere of specific places, as well as my memories of conversations and events. Using my informed imagination, I augment details and remove what is unnecessary to the story. Despite such frequent literary liberties, the story is deeply true.

*B*IRTH TO *A*GE *E*LEVEN

Dr. Menzies and Me

Dr. Adam Menzies of Morden, Manitoba held me by my ankles and gave me a gentle shake until I cried out. "Aha, Mrs. Neufeld," he said to my mother. "Another little Mennonite devil!" He chuckled and handed me to the nurse. She cleaned and wrapped me. Mama, lying back on the bed, smiled. The nurse settled me against my mother, who mouthed a quiet prayer of thanks for a thirteenth child to love. She looked at my face to see whom I resembled and snuggled me closer to her body. Whether a little Mennonite, a little devil, or both, it was March 4, 1939 – I had arrived, and my mama was very happy.

My life began in 1939 – and it was also the year the Second World War started. The first of these beginnings would be filled with private struggles, the second heavy with hostilities. The first was animated with life, the other replete with death. With the first driven by intrinsic life forces, the second by outside extremities, neither was predictable.

To be human is to be caught in the uneven texture of life. My years were to be filled high with both joy and unhappiness, my life much like that of any typical man in our Western culture. In fact, the intensity of personal pleasure has been mine, as have the depths of grief. Talents were meted out, and personality traits singularly endowed. In the final analysis, though, the particularities of my human living have been unique simply because they are mine.

Infant Imagining

Obviously, I remember nothing about the years immediately after I emerged into my family's world, but Mama told me about this. Somebody took me home from the hospital, but Mama stayed there with milk fever, a nasty calcium deficiency which occurred in breast-feeding women. At home without Mama, much love and devotion surrounded my baby personality, but I imagine being equally stressed by my removal from Mama's breast as by my separation from her person. One of my five sisters, Martha, spent hours soothing me in the rocking chair while I drank from a bottle. Amply rewarded for my baby gurgles with smiles and "coo-coos" from each member of my large family, I became known as Martha's sweetheart. Everybody loved the baby, and a great deal of demonstrative affection must have swirled around me. But I'm sure I really missed my mama.

She came home a few weeks later and, although I remained limited to the bottle, I marvel at how deeply Mama's intensive baby-care must have stimulated my consciousness as I began to grasp my separateness. "*Hen*-ry," she said, gently poking my chest. "*Hen*-ry." She directed her finger to herself and said, "*Ma*-ma." She repeated this many times daily, she told me later, and after a while I began to sort things out – my first tentative attempt to know my*self*.

My Mother's Character

How a mature brain can visualize its own existence is a mystery. How a child's brain sees itself is even more puzzling. Despite this, I remember childhood times when I guessed, more or less accurately, just how I fit into my family.

A little child seems capable of calculating, up to a point, its value to a group. If a home consistently affirms the child's inherent worth, the odds are high that youngsters begin to develop an appreciation for their personal value.

I learned from Mama that I was good. Even when she spanked me, my history with her assured me, at some level, that this was done for reasons unrelated to my essential worth. I could neither verbalize nor think through such a concept, but if someone else, like Papa, did precisely the same thing as Mama, I intuitively felt that I was a bad boy.

Mama loved me without reason or cause, while my brothers and sisters loved me if I met their expectations. Siblings rarely exchanged unconditional love. We earned love from each other. A new baby was born with a halo and, for a while, was the exception.

It was Mama's "no-strings-attached" love that gave me whatever steadiness of self-esteem I have today. The faith which I have in my *self* is directly related to the unambivalent caring she gifted me. Other people loved me, too, but it was she who laid the groundwork that allowed me to accept my*self* without stumbling over drastic reservations such as those that bedevilled Papa.

My self-acceptance is not a solid fixture. It falters. Neither do I function with consistent confidence. In a crunch, though, I recognize my innate value as a human being. Mama and I had no issues unresolved, no necessary words unspoken. Our mutual love was palpable and unabashed. Mama had everything to do with that.

A long list of positive adjectives is required to describe Mama, an unsophisticated and largely unschooled woman. She had an extremely difficult life. Catastrophically, she buried five of her thirteen children. Although her husband gave his whole life to physically sustain his family, he was most difficult to live with. She lived in an era when women accepted their tough, unfair roles with a forgiving silence.

Although she had many reasons to reach the end of her life unhappy and unfulfilled, Mama died a gracious and kind woman, with a child-like and unswerving faith in her God.

Mama and Papa and Families Leave Russia

Mama, whose given names were Katerina Linda, was born in Russia at the turn of the twentieth century. H. H. Klassen, her father, was a wealthy Mennonite owner of four flour mills, who sent little Katerina and her siblings to a private Mennonite school. Unfortunately, a country-wide revolution soon forced the children to stay home. This well-monied family subsequently lived through the brutality of a revolution which, among many worse brutalities, left them destitute.

After his last mill was confiscated in the mid 1920s, my strong-willed grandfather decided the family would leave its motherland. My mother and father, newly married, decided to join her family. Plans to emigrate to Canada began.

Leaving close relatives and good friends behind was dreadful. The girls and women cried all the time, while the men waited until they were alone in the barn before they blew their noses. There were no viable alternatives to emigrating, even though those who stayed behind did so with the knowledge they would never see their emigrating loved ones again. They would be gone until meeting in heaven.

One night, the large Klassen family, my mama and papa included, hitched their four best horses to their best and biggest wagon and headed for the Black Sea. Here the newly established Mennonite Central Committee (Canada) had arranged to financially assist them in their trip across the ocean.

After a horrid voyage, the family reached Canada, a country full of great empty spaces waiting for immigrants to fill the land with peace – and wheat. For most Mennonite immigrants like Mama's siblings, Canada proved to be remarkably compatible with their physical and spiritual needs.

Papa

Peter J. Neufeld, born in 1892, grew up in Chortiza, a Mennonite village in southern Russia. His parents were landless and poor to the point of serious deprivation. When he was nine, his mother died of typhoid fever; his father was killed in an accident several months later. A pre-revolutionary government divvied up Papa's eight sisters and brothers as it saw fit. My father was sent to a government-run school.

He showed considerable mathematical talent, and in 1915, shortly before the Russian Revolution, Peter Neufeld graduated with twelve years of schooling, academically prepared to work as an accountant. After his studies, he was employed in that capacity by a co-op store.

My father and my mother met soon after, and their many years together began with a series of monumental life changes.

Life taught Papa that he was undeserving. Often, I heard him say, "*Ich bin so schlecht*" [I am so bad]. As I grew older, I recognized that his belief in himself was seriously diminished. His self-derogatory comments echoed painfully into Canada's vast spaces and, inevitably, left a negative imprint on my own self-esteem.

I was a grown man before I understood just how profoundly his stressful childhood impinged on the rest of his life. How devastated he must have been when his father died in an accident six months after his mother succumbed to typhoid fever. What a dreadful rupture must have sliced down the centre of his boyhood! After he lost all but one sibling to the slaughtering of violent gangs, he was placed into a government-adoptive situation, and subsequently spent years attending a state-controlled school. His bad fortune lightened as he developed into a capable student with a special aptitude in mathematics. No magic, however, healed his self-abnegation. Respect for his *self,* as one whom God loved, was frightfully fragile, or absent altogether.

Immigrating to Canada did not alter Papa's setbacks. When he applied for an accountancy job in Morden, Manitoba, business owners on Main Street scoffed: "An immigrant accountant? Hah!" Rather than succeed because of his hard-earned expertise from Russian schools, he was handed a spade and sent to turn over the soil in a rich man's vegetable garden. His unschooled brothers-in-law, conversely, bought hundreds of acres of productive soil for a handful of change per acre. They achieved financial comfort relatively soon, while my landless papa spaded on.

In the first half of the twentieth century spankings were common among both Mennonites and non-Mennonites. Papa gave me what I, hyperbolically, called beatings. Almost worse than the pain were his predictable apologies the next day. I cried at the first event, but he cried at both.

Papa used his belt and hit me hard. The violence frightened me, but I wanted very badly not to blame him. He must be tired from work, I told myself, and being regularly turned down by Morden's businessmen who mocked his Russian accounting certificate would make anybody angry.

Once, I went swimming instead of getting some eggs for Mama from our henhouse. She told Papa, and he promptly pointed to our empty living room. Once there, he said, "Kneel." I knelt over one of the chairs we used for daily family devotions, and he whacked me four times. I cried out and could not hold back my tears. He wept quietly and put his belt back on. I smelled his sweat. A few days later, the children at school laughed when I scratched at the scabs through my pants.

The next day Papa asked me to forgive him for hitting me so hard. I was quiet for a few seconds. I felt confused about his routine apologies, but when he started to tear up, I hurriedly said, "Yes, yes, of course," and he gave me a hug and left.

A few weeks later, I thought Papa had gone to work. To be doubly safe I lowered the family radio's volume and held it next to my ear. If Papa ever heard me listening to *The Lone Ranger* I would be in serious trouble – but there he was standing right behind me. I think, now, he meant to strike the radio, but his fist struck the side of my head just over my right ear. I fell to the floor beside the pump organ with pieces of broken radio around me.

"You tried to deceive me!" he shouted. It was true – he had said there must be no more listening to violent radio programs like *The Lone Ranger*. I lay on the floor not feeling much at all, just shock. Papa said, "Get up," and pointed to the organ bench before taking off his belt. The pain hurt more than normally, but for the first time I managed not to cry – but he began to cry before he left the room.

The severe headache I got that afternoon made me angry. Over time, a revelation dawned: not I, but Papa should be ashamed. The excuses I had been making for his violence didn't ring true anymore.

The next day we met halfway up the stairs and he put out a hand to stop me, and I heard him swallow. He said, *"Ich bin so schlecht"* [I am so bad] and wiped his cheeks with his fingertips. "Will you forgive me?"

"Yes," I said automatically.

"Come, sit with me," Papa said, and we walked downstairs to the living room. He wiped his eyes again and pulled me close to him as we sat on the couch. He took a deep breath and said, "In the Bible, King David did very bad things. Yet he was called a man close to the heart of God." Papa took another deep breath and looked at me more calmly. "Do you know why God forgave him each time?"

I looked at the small, framed picture of *The Blue Boy* hanging on the wall and shook my head. "King David always repented," Papa said. "He always asked for forgiveness, and that's what saved him from God's wrath." I stared at the Blue Boy's fancy clothes that made him look like a girl, and I didn't like him anymore. "Therefore, you must forgive me, too." Papa glanced at the clock on the wall. "I'm late!" he said and rushed out of the room, the screen door banging behind him.

The gash was mostly hidden among my hair, but blood dribbled from above my ear and down the left side of my neck. I wiped at it with the back of my hand and tried to hide the injury by carefully doing a comb-over with my fingers. My thoughts were mixed, but then I noticed *The Blue Boy*. I told myself, "Someday, I'll take that stupid *Blue Boy* and smash it on a very big rock."

Papa lived his life switching from one end of his emotional continuum to the other, spreading from anger to generosity, from bitterness to amiability.

In church, Papa impressed people with his skill as a reciter. The narrative poems he recited were usually fifteen minutes long, and he presented them from memory. Papa knew how to hold an audience, and the congregation sat perfectly still, thoroughly engaged. He reached deeply into his heart, and when the narrative approached an emotional climax, Papa sometimes stopped to cry. He pulled out a white handkerchief, wiped his eyes, blew his nose, regained his composure and went on. Both embarrassed and proud, his listening children kept their heads down. Deeply moved by the dramatic storyline and by Papa's emotional involvement, not a few listeners wept along with him. I postponed my crying until bedtime.

When church was over Sunday at noon, Papa scurried into the lobby to assist other men in putting on their overcoats. Papa did this so regularly that he recognized each man's outside apparel hanging on a hook and had the coat ready and open for each smiling male member of our congregation. When they thanked him, he told them he was their servant.

Papa was a complicated person. Whether motivated by concern for others or by his personal sense of worthlessness, he always stood ready to help. Parallel to his generosity was his fastidious honesty. "A promise made is a debt unpaid," he once told me. His integrity was his trademark.

Despite the various hurts he caused me, I recognized Papa's multiple assets. I felt proud of his scholarly grasp of three languages, his literary activities (public recitations and private reading), his generosity, his dogged endurance, his well-known hospitality and his deep bass singing voice. Papa's remarkable memory, his mathematical skills, his impeccable handwriting, and his faultless German grammar had made him into a fine scholar. His respect for education and his pride in his children's success was a big factor in their accomplishments. He had an easy capacity for making friends, and his subsequent loyalty was commendable. His sense of responsibility to those poorer than he was demonstrated by his over-giving. Perhaps most noteworthy was that Papa's day-after-day commitment to his family's welfare, even when he felt angry and unloving, never failed him.

At work, he volunteered for the most physically challenging jobs. Whether he unloaded a trailer filled with gravel on a road construction site or scrubbed the floor of a rich man's largest room, Papa never stopped until the job was completed. Taking a break was time lost. At the workday's end, Papa chopped an enormous supply of wood for our cookstove. No one worked harder than Papa.

Papa once saved my life. Before I was one, pneumonia, a killer in 1940, took over my tiny lungs and I was rushed to the hospital. Doctors did what they could, but finally told my parents I would die because of the extreme dehydration that consumed me. Much later Mama told me they had no needles small enough to put me on intravenous.

Papa, who worked as a caretaker in the building, was told the news, and he hurried to my tiny hospital crib. "He can't drink," the nurse told him. With a decisiveness quite unlike him, Papa asked for the smallest spoon available and a glass of water. All night long he coaxed and pushed cool water between my cracked baby lips. In the morning, surprised doctors found me improving – and I lived.

Papa and Me and Ice Cream

The morning after my conversion to Jesus, Papa put on his cap and said to me, "Come."

"Where to?" I asked, but he said nothing. I felt excited and a little nervous. I unhooked my cap from a nail in the wall and followed him outside. "What did I do wrong?"

"Nothing's wrong." Papa seemed strangely composed. He didn't act angry, but his mood didn't seem especially happy, either. I couldn't tell what to expect.

Papa stood five feet nine inches tall and weighed only one hundred and forty-five pounds, but he walked like a soldier: upright and quickly. I half-ran beside him, and his big hand around my little one felt warm. I started to chatter but he paid no attention, so I grew silent as well.

We walked on a sidewalk with rotting boards. As we got closer to the stores, the old boards were replaced with shiny new ones. Once uptown, the sidewalk turned to concrete so smooth that I wished I owned a bicycle.

When we met people, I noticed how politely Papa greeted them. He said "Good morning" to everyone. For one man he also touched his cap, and a little later said to me, "That was Mr. Crosly who owns

East End Grocery." A man with a white collar approached us and Papa touched his cap and said, "Good morning." He waited until the man couldn't hear, and then he said, "That was the United Church minister." He bowed to a fat man smoking a cigar, touched his cap, and greeted him as well. "The mayor of Morden," he whispered. We met a group of men with lunch kits and he said, "Good morning," but didn't touch his cap.

Papa steered me through the door of a shop marked Goodie's Confectionary. "What's this?" I asked.

"You'll see," he said, and chose a booth. I slid next to him and he said, "No, no, sit across from me," and I scrambled to the other side.

I stared at the shiny tabletops and the stools which looked like short soldiers standing in a row. I supposed this was a restaurant. It certainly smelled like food.

A girl dressed like a nurse came to our booth and asked, "What'll ya have?"

"Please, two vanilla ice cream cones," said Papa. The girl walked quickly behind the counter and, with a large spoon, scraped at one of the round cardboard boxes. I could hear the ice cream scraper dragging across the inside of the box. She pushed the ice cream deep into each cone. Reaching back into the vanilla box, she refilled the ladle and worked these second mounds of ice cream on top of the first ones. Finally, she half-ran back to us and handed one to Papa and one to me.

"There y'are," she said. She took the two five-cent pieces Papa handed her and hurried to the next customer.

My eyes popped. There was so much ice cream it almost fell off the top. I knew that in Canada, Papa had never earned more than a pittance. When my five oldest siblings had moved away to work or

16

go on to school, some of them sent a portion of their earnings home. Today only Helen and Emma and I remained, and while Mama and Papa were slightly less poor now, spending a dime on ice cream had never happened in my life.

"Don't gawk," said Papa. "Eat it."

"Without a spoon?" I asked, and Papa's lips twitched.

"Watch me," he said.

"Don't we have to give thanks?" I asked.

"Not just for ice cream," Papa said. "Watch me."

He licked at his frozen ice cream, and licked it again. I did as well, and soon I was licking as fast as I could to keep the melting ice cream from running down the side. It reminded me of snow but sweet and full of a flavour I'd never tasted. "Oh, my!" I said.

"Your chin's dripping." Papa reached across the table with his red handkerchief. I wiped my mouth with it. He used his teeth to bite little bits of ice cream from the top. Except for the sounds he made, I copied him and soon we were both down to where the yellow cones started. Papa looked at me, and once more his lips twitched with pleasure.

Returning a Dime

I had some awful phobias, but that didn't mean other people in our family weren't suffering from their own extreme character traits.

Years later at Papa's funeral, Preacher Friesen reminded the congregation that Brother Neufeld was a giving man. In fact, he said, overly so. People in the pews nodded and smiled. Everyone knew about the irony in this poor man's extravagance. Papa stood so eager to help, I felt embarrassed by his willingness to belittle himself in the process.

Sitting in the church pew that funeral day, I remembered the morning Papa came home from work looking like his usual worn-out self. He said hello to Mama and me and hung his cap on a nail in the wall. He put a brown bag of eggs on the table where I was doing my Grade Ten homework.

Papa pulled a few coins from his pocket, and counted them. "Oh, my!" he said. "The clerk gave me back ten cents too much." He jumped up, grabbed his cap and half ran through the outside door.

I was startled by his agitated departure. "What happened? Where's Papa going?" I asked Mama.

Mama pounded her big hunk of bread dough a hard couple of punches. "Back up town to give the dime back to the clerk," she said. "He shouldn't be so hard on himself. He's already so tired." She came over to the table and picked up the bag of eggs.

In my mind I could smell the bread that Mama would have ready by suppertime. I said, "Why doesn't he pay it back tomorrow?"

Mama sighed. "Because," she said, "it's a matter of honour with him. He wouldn't be able to sleep with that on his mind."

"A dime?" I asked. "A dime, and he can't sleep?"

"A dime," Mama agreed. "A dime, and he can't sleep." She sighed.

Concern about Papa's tiredness after walking extra miles because of a dime tugged at me. "When do you think he'll be back, Mama?" I asked.

"I'm not sure," she said. "We'll have to wait and see. Just do your schoolwork and don't worry too much."

I bent my head back to my books, but I worried about Papa even though Mama said not to.

Papa's *Seelenangst*

On occasion, Papa's uncertainty about his personal salvation gripped him terribly, and he was overcome by *Seelenangst* (intense fear that he would be condemned as *schlecht*, or bad on Judgment Day). During such anxiety attacks, he would sweat profusely, be frightened to the point of whimpering, afraid that his pounding heart would accelerate out of control and he would die. Mama sent one of us for Preacher Friesen who hurried over to settle Papa. I listened to them on the floor of my room through the stovepipe hole which was empty in summer.

Preacher Friesen reviewed the fundamentals of salvation: we are born in sin, but if we ask Jesus to forgive us our sins, His death ensures Heaven. He said, "Only believe." With a hand on Papa's shoulder, he asked God to comfort Brother Peter. He asked that Papa be able to accept God's unbreakable promise. Silence spread. I heard the sparrows' staccato chattering, and the curtains lifting in the breeze.

Papa knelt and prayed. His tremulous voice admitted his many sins, and he thanked God for interceding. His voice broke. "Amen," Preacher Friesen said. "Brother Peter, you are, like me, a sinner, but we are not bad men." He helped Papa to his feet and shook his hand. Then he gave him a long man-to-man hug and left the room.

I slipped from my bedroom to the girls' room across the hall where the window was open, and I overheard Preacher Friesen wishing Mama well. Then he asked, "Where is your Henry?"

"Oh, playing somewhere," Mama said, leaning on her hoe. She smiled at him. "Many thanks," she said.

Preacher Friesen lifted his hand in acknowledgement and said, "Your boy has promise. Wish him well from me." He slid easily into his black '52 Chrysler and drove away. Mama laid down her hoe and hurried to the house.

The Orange

One Saturday afternoon, Mama sent me upstairs to have a nap. I sneaked back to see what she and Marion were up to.

"Mama, can I please have an orange?" asked my fifteen-year-old sister Marion. Mama was the Keeper of all Christmas-To-Come items. She even kept track of the exact number of fruits we had in the cellar. Marion wanted an orange so much she felt extra spit in her mouth.

"Oh, no, Marion," said Mama. "We have to keep them for Christmas."

Marion used her method for all things hard to get. "Pleeeeze, Mama? Pleeeeze!"

"Well, I suppose one or two may have begun to rot. If you find an orange that has started to go bad, you can cut away the rotten part and eat the rest. But if they are all good, then I'll have to say no."

"Oh, goody!" Marion looked down to the cellar door built into the floor and tried to lift it by using the iron ring. She couldn't. Mama left the potatoes she was peeling and, using only two fingers, pulled at the loop trying to raise the cellar door. She jerked at the ring until the hinges squeaked, and the door moved a little. Moving her feet further apart, Mama lifted hard until it rose all the way. She laid it on its back and looked at the ancient steps leading into the darkness.

She said, "Don't fall, child. And remember how low the ceiling is." Then she laughed at what she had said about the ceiling: Marion was still so short. Marion inched down the steps and stood at the bottom.

"I'm scared," she said. "Everything's black. I can't see a single thing." She shivered. "And it's cold."

"I know where the oranges are," said Mama. "I can find them in the dark." She stepped cautiously down the rotting stairs, brushed past Marion and took a few steps into the cellar. "Here's the box," she said. "Now up you go."

Marion scurried up the stairs, sat on the kitchen floor and dangled her legs into the cellar. Mama climbed up a few steps and set the box on the floor. The cardboard box had been opened by someone with a hammer claw, so Mama jerked at the thin top boards and together they looked in. The cool oranges looked shiny and edible.

"They're so terribly beautiful!" gasped Marion. She lifted a few so she could see the bottom row. "There are no rotten ones, Mama. I couldn't have a good one, could I? Just one?" She looked hopefully at Mama who shook her head, closed the box and returned it to the shelf.

"Three weeks till Christmas," Mama said. "We'll eat them together, not one at a time." From where she stood, her head was level with Marion's waist. Impulsively she put her arms around her daughter's legs and hugged them. Her voice broke when she said, "Thirteen years old and already you have the legs of a woman!"

Marion pulled away. "Oh, Mama, you shouldn't talk like that," she said, then jumped up, and ran upstairs.

Mama stood still in the silence. She closed her eyes. "Lord, please keep her safe," she whispered. Then she smiled to herself and added, "Pleeeeze!" Mama climbed the remaining steps and searched for the door's iron ring. She placed two fingers into the ring and lowered the door until it lay even and strong in its groove.

Swinging

Ten giant steps from the broken screen door of our house stood an ash tree so high its leaves waved in the sky. Twenty feet above its base, huge branches jutted out from its trunk.

My brother Jack brought home a rope and a borrowed ladder. Using a board from our junk pile and our ancient saw, he cut out a swing seat. Then he twisted his all-purpose knife round and round and meticulously carved out two circular holes and drew the rope through both. He leaned the ladder against the thick branch, climbed up and tied the ropes tightly around the branch, and a swing was born. I watched in young amazement.

Jack turned to me. "Want a ride?"

I said, "Yes, yes!" and slipped onto the board. "But not too hard!"

"I didn't build it for sissies," Jack said, and laughed. He stood behind me and, with his hands on the two ropes, began to push. He pushed gently at first, but as the long rope increased the speed of my gliding back and forth, he leaned into me harder and harder. Finally, he ran under the swing and gave my butt a final shove. I rose like a bird, and each time I reached the swing's maximum height, I hovered for an instant on the apex of the swing – and smoothly retreated into the flying arc.

"I love it!" I shouted. "Push me higher!"

Mama called through the window, "Not so hard! He might fall!" Jack eased up, and gradually my half-loop slowed and stopped.

I felt as though I had reached a summit, a spire, an apogee of sorts. I slid off the wooden seat and looked at Jack. He grinned and ruffled my hair.

Henry's Death and Funeral

Papa told me once that Mama had a second baby boy in the mid-1930s. They named him Henry, a name which I inherited years later. After Henry turned four, he was hospitalized with *Knochenfraß*, or bone cancer. The doctor diagnosed the disease as terminal and sent the three of them home. Mama and Papa, in a state of shock, cried, but the reality of the doctor's prognosis was much too dreadful to absorb at one telling.

The Peter J. Neufeld family was poor. Many immigrants had a hard time finding work, and Papa was one of them. He helped Mama as Henry's health worsened. Papa rocked him continually during Henry's waking hours for the next thirty days.

Their tiny house was miserably inadequate, but the rent was cheap. They managed with two upstairs bedrooms, a downstairs kitchen where they ate their meals, and one other room that served as a living room and sleeping quarters for the oldest girls. A rocking chair, older than the house, helped soothe each baby as it arrived.

Mama planted a small garden. Potatoes and carrots stored in the cool basement went a long way to cover their food needs. With Papa being unemployed, they ate potatoes twice a day instead of the usual once. Someone kind brought them a sack of flour, a literal lifesaver. Every room had the odour of cooking, a fresh, familiar smell.

Henry slept in the quiet, tidy basement. One night the little boy's breathing degenerated into irregular gasping, and he died. Our parents watched, listening to Henry's last short breath – a tiny intake of air with no exhalation. They stared at the dead little boy. Copious tears, like rivulets flowing down a small slope after a thunderstorm, streamed down their cheeks in a rush. They struggled not to be heard by their sleeping children, but their grief proved impossible to constrain.

Papa roused himself and nailed together a few boards he found in the yard. He built a crude little box with a light plywood top. Twice he struck his thumb. Mama held Henry, her eyes drinking in the last image of her still-warm son. Her quiet weeping was continuous.

After a time, Mama chose their best second-hand blanket, swaddled Henry, and laid him into his final bed. They both prayed over Henry's body, struggling to make themselves understood to each other as well as to their Maker. Their prayers were an embodiment of faith in an inscrutable God whom they tried to trust even in this moment of inexplicable dying. A sense of unreality overcame them. Like a fog lifting in the candle-lit basement, their initial sense of disbelief eventually shifted, and they began moving towards an acknowledgement that another child was dead.

One of the children called from upstairs, and the parents pulled themselves away from their silent son and relinquished him to the cellar. Mama stumbled slightly on the stairs as she looked back over her shoulder to ensure that Henry was properly covered.

A week earlier, the family had been quarantined with scarlet fever, so Papa went out the back door and called their neighbours. Someone heard, and he asked them to let their minister know about Henry's death. Strict rules forbad entry into their house, but arrangements would be made for a funeral service to be held the following day, outside their house, in the yard.

The next morning, friends and relatives gathered on the outside of the fence surrounding the Neufelds' yard. Papa carried the home-made coffin outside, where he tilted it so that people could catch a glimpse of four-year-old Henry's face. The parents and oldest children stood beside the coffin, while the youngest looked through the windows. They could hear little of what was said by the minister, but they could see their dead brother's face and hear the sad singing of the people lining the fence.

When the service was over, Papa placed the lid on the coffin and nailed it shut with tiny nails, the hammer blows painfully at odds with the hushed surroundings. The town policeman came into the yard and Papa gently lifted the homemade box and yielded it to the officer who carried it to his car. With great care he placed it on the front seat where he could see it, and drove Henry to the town cemetery. Henry was buried in a grave marked only by a small wooden cross.

As they left, the people waved to the family, and a number of them cried out words of comfort. Mama gestured to the children and the family. Managing without a single touch of comfort, they walked into their home. Some relatives remained outside the fence as though events were not yet finished, but eventually everyone left. Everything was quite finished.

Someone had told Papa that there was work available in the adjacent town. Never failing to jump at employment of any kind, he hastily kissed each of his children goodbye, nodded towards Mama, but because the children were watching, he did not kiss her. He hurriedly changed his clothes for the seven-mile walk. In the street he looked for a vehicle heading in the direction he was going, but everyone had left.

As he neared the outskirts of his hometown, he began to weep. He had no idea when he would be coming home, or where he would sleep that night.

Mama, alone with the children, sat down at the empty table and sighed. She was very tired, very sad. The children felt the day's solemnity and played quietly. Mama put her arms on the table, her head on her arms, and wept quietly.

Somewhere between praying and napping and weeping, Mama heard scrabbling sounds coming from the roof. Still crying, she walked outside to see. On each corner of the roof, she saw four boy angels. She stopped crying. Wonderfully moved, she looked again, and they were gone. "*Ich danke dir, lieber Gott,*" Mama prayed. She repeatedly thanked God for this wonderful manifestation of caring. Back in the house, she assumed the physical and spiritual positions she had left a few minutes ago. The children had no immediate needs, and she fell asleep at the table.

Much later she woke, calm and somewhat refreshed. The assurance that she would someday, somehow, see little Henry again comforted her. A growing serenity suffused her as she got up from her chair, put her children to bed, and kissed them goodnight. Except for her ponderings about the boy angels standing on the four corners of the roof, and worrying about Papa, a certain normality and routine had returned to her life.

The West End

I was my parents' last child and still in my infancy when Mama and Papa, my seven siblings and I moved to Morden, a small town of eighteen hundred people in southern Manitoba. Papa never found work geared to his best abilities, but he rented a small house in town, a shack that sat next to a farm-like dugout. In a heavy rain, the dugout overflowed, and water almost reached our backyard. Jack called our place "the hut beside the dugout." The open water bred at least ten million mosquitoes annually.

I was six, and the Second World War was over. A spurt in Canada's economy enabled Papa to borrow money from some well-to-do Mennonite church members, and suddenly we owned a house in Morden's West End. It wasn't paid for, of course – not even a down payment – but Jack said that technically it was ours, and anyway, the monthly payments cost less than renting. Even if the building turned out to be less than we hoped for, at least we'd have more bedrooms.

Uncle Willie, Mama's generous brother, arrived before noon. His single-cylinder John Deere tractor pulled a bare-bones hayrack. The outfit made enough noise to scare the gophers behind our shack into their burrows. Unsupervised, we children loaded household belongings haphazardly. Personal belongings got thrown on last.

All the girls thought the rack looked ugly. Old dressers were tied to the hayrack's end boards with binder twine; the drawers, unfastened, had slid open and girls' underwear hung out and waved in the wind. We fastened pieces of beds and ancient mattresses to the wooden floor. Mama had previously poured the kerosene from our lamps into a leak-proof can and wrapped the glass cylinders in bedclothes. Our one table had been dismantled and its boards tied lengthwise to the hayrack's sides. We piled chairs on top of chairs, upside down. An assemblage of ten people's clothing was crammed, like loose handkerchiefs, into the various spaces generated by our household goods.

Eventually, everyone jumped onto the hayrack, Uncle Willie carefully let out the clutch of the John Deere, and we were off. While the girls hid their faces from passing cars, I was too young for self-consciousness. I loved getting a ride behind the tractor and shouted and raised a hand to everybody who stared at us.

"Don't wave!" hissed Marion, but I was six years old and didn't understand her reluctance to be seen. If anyone doubted how poor we were, there was no hiding it now. The whole contraption made a strange and wild sight.

We drove through the West End and saw our new horrid-looking house before we saw Papa and Jack. Martha yelled, "Ugly!"

The original clapboard had been unpainted for so long, evidence of any colour had disappeared and given way to a dirty grey dullness. The house was one-and-a-half stories high and resembled a miniature grain elevator leaning, with the wind, toward the southeast. A narrow building, it looked even smaller than the shack we had just left. Broken chimney bricks lay scattered on the roof. Eavestroughs had never existed and, running off the roof, the rains had etched a six-inch miniature ditch in the earth surrounding the house. The four crooked windows in the east wall reminded me of crossed eyes staring at each other. A shed was attached to the house's west end. Its roof sloped at a crooked angle as though bolstered up by two men, one tall and one the height of a young boy. We hadn't anticipated a mansion, but this was a disaster.

None of us noticed the good things: a huge yard and dozens of leafy maples and elms and ash trees stretching up and out. Even the magnificence of the trees could not lift our spirits. We were blinded to the yard's beauty by our disappointment in the ugly house. The anticipated fun of moving day had petered out.

Jack came over to Mama and me and said, "The outside looks like an old barn for old cows, but let's go look inside."

"I'm not going in," I said, but Mama grasped my hand and led the Neufeld procession through the torn screen door. Papa had been watching us, and now walked quickly away into the wooded area behind the yard.

In the shed, torn pieces of linoleum were held down by nails so small their heads had torn through. Under the linoleum, the floor looked cracked and dried out from the extremes of temperature. The windows allowed for lots of light, but two of them were cracked and one was broken, with a piece of cardboard flapping in the empty space. The inside walls were painted a greyish white but the narrow boards running up and down were old-fashioned, narrow and dry. Except for the absence of manure, I thought, abandoned barns likely smelled like this: musky, and past the time to be torn down.

Jack examined a spot on the wall where a splinter of wood had fallen away. He looked into the wall and said, "No insulation."

A summer bake oven stood near the chimney which reached through the roof. Somebody ambitious had recently polished the stovepipes. Stretching from the stove to the chimney, they were such a shiny black that the contrast made this corner of the room look like an item from the newspaper funnies.

I jerked open the door under the sink and found a pail half-full of used water. A piece of soap lay on the cupboard, and Mama picked it up. "Homemade," she said, and laid it back.

"What's that on the ceiling?" asked Helen.

"Water marks," said Mama. "The ceiling leaks."

We had moved to the only part of town with its own name: West End. Morden had no East End, or South End, or North End – only the West End. A preliminary attraction for me was the Dead Horse Creek which flooded each spring, overnight. Homeowners hated the creek's sudden runover, but we boys loved the excitement and potential danger a flash flood carried. Another Morden thrill was our close-up view of enormous steam-powered locomotives that stopped to "fill 'er up" at the Canadian Pacific Railway's water tower, a block from our house.

The West End offered many secondary sources of excitement. If you owned a cow, you were allowed to let it graze on town property near your house. Some people raised hens and a few roosters; one year we raised some pigs with no complaints from neighbours. Few residents owned cars and so summer dust was light, the air as clear as in the country. We found much to love in Morden's West End.

Jack Rebuilding with Brick Siding

We tried many ways to keep winter drafts out of our house. Pink insulation placed on the inside bottom of windows helped. Around each inside hall window, where windows were less conspicuous, we taped large sheets of plastic. Freezing winter nights, we rolled up pieces of rug in the evening and jammed them lengthwise in the crack where the door met the floor, even though these rug fragments were frozen stiff in the morning. Some school holidays we spent the day squeezing quick-hardening liquid plastic into cracks around light switches and electric plug-ins. We tried ingenious ways to keep out Jack Frost's sneaky drafts. We were at war.

Sometimes we played a game with the ice-cold drafts by looking for tiny breezes coming in through hidden places. Air moved where it shouldn't, but we couldn't find the cracks in the wall. We got on the floor and lit wooden matches, and after blowing them out, we waved them back and forth so that the moving smoke would show us where the cold air was coming in. This never worked, although we could feel tiny wisps of icy air slipping in around the baseboards.

Then Jack found the answer. Most of the air seemed to be moving right through the uninsulated walls themselves. Jack heard of a new product called brick siding which was overlapped and tacked to the outside of houses. It should work perfectly.

One Saturday in autumn, Jack brought home a sample from The Morden Lumber Yard in which Preacher Friesen was a partner. Brick siding, a tar-like product that came in heavy, two-foot-wide rolls, needed to be flattened against the outside of a house with thick, long tacks. We tried some of the material on the chicken house, and when that worked, Jack ordered a truckload. Our house exterior was made of rough boards, so we didn't have to do a stud search for wooden two-by-fours. Jack lined up a few rolls, and Helen, Emma, and I, the three youngest children, nailed them on. For the first time I found that physical work could be fun.

Jack financed the project with money he earned working after school at Cochlan's Department Store, and Preacher Friesen, who owned half of The Morden Lumber Yard, always agreed to low monthly payments. For reasons never explained but somehow understood, The Morden Lumber Yard cancelled Jack's last few monthly payments.

The Island

As poor as any family in town, we were rich in trees which covered the two acres of land that came with the house. The Dead Horse Creek ran directly behind our property. I named the place where an offshoot of the creek flowed around our land in spring, and dried up in summer The Island. The proximity of these little woods to our house, as well as my proclivity for drama, made possible my first reflective appreciation of nature and its relationship to what I later came to call sacred.

I learned quickly to treasure this space of wonderment. Dozens of trees dominated The Island, and uncultivated flowers bloomed in hidden places. High branches swayed lightly in the tiny breeze, and mysterious shadows moved over the ground. Where sunlight penetrated the crowns of trees, low grass grew in bunches.

The area was isolated and private. "It's mine," I thought. "Nobody comes here." At six, I was too young to articulate my feelings, but I was pious even then, and whispered a prayer of thanks. My father owned this mini forest; I would be the one shaped by it.

Up to now, family and church were the most influential entities in my life, but as the clock ticked, this island of quietness became my most treasured haven. I felt the wind's gentleness on my skin, and my eyes spotted countless shades of green. Like an opened umbrella, a cloud shadowed my secret spot. I touched the leaf of a tree between my lips and fingered its delicate skin. I recognized the presence of something I could not name but which made me feel safe and happy.

Dead Horse Creek flowed by my feet, rippling slightly. The sun had dried the debris left by the flash flood in spring, and dried branches lay washed up on the banks. We were rich in trees, and our future swimming hole, deep and clear, would have been a few feet of tepid water if not for the beaver dam further up the creek. I hoped for rain, if only to see the water trickle over the dam.

Much later, I kept a list of birds in my new forest. Bluejays, meadowlarks, robins, red-winged blackbirds, bobolinks, orioles, mourning doves, crows, finches, sparrows, woodpeckers, kingfishers, and water birds such as geese, mallards, wood ducks, cranes, waterhens and a variety of other birds I could not name, were everywhere I looked.

Morden was still a young town. The Second World War, just ended, impacted us not at all, and although the prairie all around us was covered with fields of grain, here and there clumps of trees stood, not yet mowed down by caterpillars that seemed huge to us then, though they were little machines by today's standards. My Island was one of those one-acre places happily saved by pure accident or good fortune.

Mrs. McCulloch and Grade Four

Elementary school had a few anxieties easily outweighed by the fine times. The year 1949 created a mountain of memorable experiences because my teacher was Mrs. McCulloch. A motherly woman who ran a busy but well-controlled classroom, she addressed pupils with a long list of endearments, and never scolded. What dissatisfaction she might occasionally experience she expressed by tilting her head and using a finger to slide her glasses down her nose a half inch. She studied individual students with her kind eyes and with no aid from her eyeglasses. The only elementary schoolteacher I ever had who found it unnecessary to raise her voice in order to manage her class, she exuded warmth, cleverly.

"Tommy, you and I both know you can write much more legibly than this," she said as she waved his untidy page toward his head until his wiry hair moved. "Why don't we let your mother know that as well? Rewrite this, please, and show her both pages at next Parents' Day, OK?"

Tommy nodded. Mrs. McCulloch smiled and handed back the page. "And why not use a reinforcement sticker to repair the bottom hole of your first try so you don't lose it before your mother sees it. All right, dear?"

I felt safe in her class.

When I mentioned her to Jack, he said, "She's taught everyone in our family, and they all say she has some kind of magic." He thought for a while and then added, "Some teachers have it, and some don't."

"Have what?" I asked

Jack was finishing Grade Twelve and he already enjoyed lecturing. "I'll tell you. Some teachers bring a particular presence with them when they're in the classroom. It's a confidence in herself that the kids sense. This self-security she possesses is contagious, makes *them* feel safe and secure, too. They want to co-operate, and when that happens, the battle is won. She transfers a particular feeling that everyone likes: I'm in charge here."

I think I liked Jack most when he talked like a smart teacher who forgot how young I was.

Miss Ingram's Map

Miss Ingram didn't need to know where each of her Grade Five students lived. That's not why she gave us a special social studies assignment. She said, "The purpose of this lesson is for you to learn how to locate yourself in time and space." We stared, clueless.

"I'll tell you what 'locate yourself in time and space' means after you've got your project started." Even if she didn't need to know where we lived, we would have to show her. I liked her very much. She used hard words, but I usually knew what they meant from the words surrounding them. Miss Ingram was always pleasant but with a kind of distance I was comfortable with. She was my friendly teacher, but she wasn't my friend like Billy or Alvin. When she spoke to me, I wanted to please her more than anything.

"Draw a map," she wrote on the blackboard in her upswept handwriting. "From where you live, up to Maple Leaf School. Name every street and use a red arrow to show how you get to school every day. I want to pretend that I am going to your home all by myself."

That evening, I started drawing my map on a piece of newsprint. The pencil stub was too short, and the paper was too small, so Mama gave me a brown grocery bag which I cut into one big piece. I got stuck. I turned the bag over and started again. I got stuck again. There were many different ways to get to school and I didn't know which route Miss Ingram would want me to choose.

Sometimes I walked past the Harasymchuks' yard where the old Russian couple with the over-sized, silent collie lived. To get to the Harasymchuks', I drew an unused road between bushes that had not felt a grader in decades. I sketched the bushes on either side.

Studying the map I was drawing, I saw I could always walk through the bush if I wasn't so frightened. Jack believed fear itself was not a shameful thing; what was shameful was allowing oneself to quit. So I continued with my fourth map, which ran through the bush on the other side, where a huge German Shepherd usually lay half asleep in the shade. He seldom moved, so I kept drawing.

My hand trembled as I traced a jerky red line past the Harasymchuks' shack to the water tower next to the tracks. When my pencil stopped, my eyes closed and, in my mind, I saw a blur of brown and black race toward me. I imagined I heard a soft guttural grunt and the huge dog stopped short. He never barked, but he growled. I shook my head and jerked out of my reverie. I wouldn't be able to meet Miss Ingram's expectations at this rate, I thought, so I turned right with my pencil and traced the red colour parallel to the railway.

Here I had to decide: should I choose the secondary road running beside the tracks, or should I take the cindered way? I decided to go east and pulled my pencil onto the tracks for a long way, almost into town, and turned left after the second railroad crossing. At the mayor's house I drew my red line straight north for two blocks, over the highway and up to the front doors of Maple Leaf School. Done. I could hardly wait to show my map to the best Grade Five teacher in Manitoba.

As I walked into the classroom the next day, I silently cheered, but I felt relief mixed with disappointment as a substitute teacher walked into Miss Ingram's room just before nine o'clock. I would have to wait until Monday to hand in my map assignment, and to hear what "located in time and space" meant.

Mama's Extended Family

Even though my father came to Canada with no family of his own, he and Mama were never alone. Their immigrant landing was scarcely soft, but was made gentler by the intimate bonds of togetherness formed by my mother's large Klassen family, and by the active life of the Mennonite Brethren Church in Morden, Manitoba.

My mother had seven siblings: four of them were farmers who lived several miles outside town. Mama's other siblings lived elsewhere in Canada, except for a sister who, together with family, lived as missionaries in what at that time was called the Belgian Congo.

All our local relatives attended the Mennonite Brethren Church, which was the social centre of their lives. The five families alternated spending Sunday afternoons together at one of their homes. My mother's siblings made their living as farmers and while they started off land-rich and cash-poor, all became materially comfortable. Laborers, like Papa, often owned no vehicle and could afford virtually no luxuries.

Uncles, aunts and about twenty-five cousins routinely showed up. After a full noon meal, the youngest stayed under the care of their mothers while the rest of us hurried outside. We played at a thousand things while our parents visited until late in the afternoon when a light lunch – *Faspa* – was served. The evening church service concluded a busy day. The church parking lot was full of Dodges and Fords and Ramblers, as well as a few new Chryslers parked conspicuously near the front door.

Toward the end of the afternoon the children gathered in the hayloft, and the highlight of the day would begin. Jack told ghost stories. Already Jack was smart as a black panther is sleek. He began organizing the group by making a long, wordless sound: "W-H-O-O-O-O-O W-O-O-H-W-O-O-O O-O W H-O-O-O-O-O W-O-O-O W-W-H- O-O-W-O-W-O O-O-O-O." Everyone settled around him as he continued this ghost-like wail until all other noise was stifled. If a little kid wailed, he said in a quiet but intense voice, "Somebody take that baby to its mommy," and one of the older girls tiptoed away with the frightened youngster. Jack gave each person a subduing glance and waited for the hush to return. Then he began.

Jack knew how to hold an audience. "Children," he said, and proceeded. His narratives were different from anything we children normally heard. All of us loved to listen, even though the youngest sometimes uttered whimpers of excitement. Jack's stories were not designed to simply frighten, but the adults in the house would scarcely consider them nourishing, either. He told short tales full of nasty goblin images and bad men. He included good girls and boys, but they were always beset by fearsome, threatening creatures who knew more about the Devil and particular trespasses than good boys and girls ever should. Evil lay planted between the lines, and though subtly presented, the sense of sin was eerily present. Jack's stories were never simply bad, but neither did they picture characters whose lives were devoted to good deeds.

The most questionable stories came from Jack's wonderful imagination. Often, he made them up as he spoke. The characters were imitative of stealthy goblins and weird witches. The endings did not necessarily conclude happily, and the slang vocabulary Jack used was unfamiliar to older children. The naughty-sounding words were strangely intriguing, but the children knew better than to experiment with them later, when their parents could hear.

Jack's Contributions

When my brother Pete and my sister Kay left home, Jack took charge of a thousand things that Papa could not possibly have done. While still in high school, Jack's job at Cochlan's Department Store paid for a long list of projects related to our house and yard, but it was mainly his non-stop physical work that got things done.

By 1949, all our neighbours had electricity and telephones; we didn't have any such modern conveniences until Jack applied and paid for them. After the three youngest children joined him in putting up the brick siding, a few nasty drafts continued to blow into the house, so Jack shoved dozens of straw bales against its outside walls. They looked awful, but nobody cared because it made such a huge difference in our miserably cold house.

The next April, Jack bought insulation and spread it all over the attic. He also borrowed money somewhere and ordered twelve yellow chicks from Alvin's dad who ran a hatchery. He organized our empty chicken barn for Mama so she could raise the dozen chicks for fall slaughtering. After he had earned some more money at Cochlan's, he laid linoleum carpet on our house's ground floor and, with the few dollars left, he ordered gravel to be spread over our dirt driveway. I used to wonder what would happen if Jack ever left.

After completing Grade Ten, I rented the property behind our house (Jack paid the bill), and the next summer I had my own tomato project which he helped me organize on the two acres of Canadian Pacific Railway property behind our house. It was actually my idea, but I never would have organized the planting of two acres of tomatoes destined for our local cannery if it wasn't for Jack.

After he left for college, Jack came home weekends to work at necessities like digging a deep hole in the ground for a new out-house. And then he built an actual outhouse which, for a while, smelled like freshly cut wood. He also replaced the ancient wooden porch of our house with a concrete one.

A few years later, Jack and my brother-in-law, Bert Loewen, poured a concrete basement floor and moved the old house onto it. Jack oversaw many other projects. The things Jack did mostly ben-efitted Mama and Papa – the two people who made it possible for their very poor family to survive many desperate years. I remember hearing them thank God in their prayers for their middle son, Jacob. I thanked God for him, too

AGE TWELVE TO SEVENTEEN

My Dog

One day a stray dog wandered onto our yard. "Half collie, at least," I said out loud. I fed it some old bread from the empty kitchen. I stroked its yellow-brown fur, and it stayed near me.

"Can I keep it, Mama?" I asked when she came out to hang the laundry. "Please!"

"What would you feed it?" Mama took the clothespins out of her mouth so she could talk. "You're only twelve but you'd have to take care of it by yourself. I don't think you're ready."

"I can get free bones at the butcher's," I said, "Or guts and stuff when Uncle Willie slaughters a pig. And you sometimes have scraps of stale bread." I patted my chest and the dog jumped up and put its paws there. He licked my face.

Mama used up the last of the clothespins. "I can smell that dog from here," she said. "You can keep it for a week, and then we'll talk about it again. But it has to sleep in the empty henhouse, and that place is very cold in the winter. And you can't bring it in the house.

Ever." She put her empty basket on her arm and walked toward the house. "That's the deal," she called over her shoulder. I figured that sounded pretty fair, so I nodded.

That night I woke after midnight and put on my pants and went to the chicken barn to see if my dog was all right. When I walked into the barn, he whined, and I whispered "Shh!" He came running to me and I fell to my knees and patted him behind his forehead and all over his back. "Quiet, shh," I said, and he settled right down, but whined a little. "Shh," I said again, and when I pushed his rump down, he lay on the straw. Already I loved that dog. I loved him with all my heart – and with my hands, and my arms, and my voice, and I would love him even more if I had something else to offer.

Back in bed I remembered how he had responded when I said, "Shh." That'll be his name, I thought, I'll call him Shh. Might sound stupid to my sisters, but he obeyed me when I called him that. Yeah, Shh.

The next day I found an old rope in the chicken barn and, using it as a leash, we walked uptown to the butcher shop. I tied Shh to a telephone post and said, "Sit." He stood there, not understanding. So, I said, "Stand!" and he stayed up quite nicely. I knew I was fooling myself, but I was pleased. He just might be a smart dog that hadn't gone to school. Like my uncles.

The butcher liked kids; he gave me a small sack of bones. "They're fresh," he said. "From a cow I butchered this morning. Your dog will gnaw at them for a week. And there's even some meat on a couple." I thanked him, and he smiled.

Outside, I untied my dog and he sniffed eagerly at the bag of bones I was holding. "They're all yours," I said, "but not yet." We ran most of the way home. In the chicken barn I gave him a bone and hooked the sack on a nail where he couldn't reach it.

The previous owner had left some ancient straw lying around. I piled the musty-smelling mess in a corner and called the dog. He was gnawing at his bone and ignored me. When I reached to take away his bone, he growled. I distracted him by waving the sack over his head. He looked up, and I snatched his bone, hung up the sack and waved his bone. Then I walked over to his straw bed, and called, "Come, Shh," and he came and stood on his straw nest trying to reach the bone.

"Down," I said, and pressed on his rump until he lay down. He grabbed the bone and began gnawing. I said, "You'll be trained soon, Shh. Now stay." He ignored me, but he stayed. "Good. See you later."

Once outside I made sure the latch on the door was tight. I looked through the dirty chicken barn windows and watched him lying on the floor, chewing. I double-checked the latch and wished I had a lock.

Winter was a challenge just trying to keep Shh properly fed and watered. The old chicken barn, where he slept and spent most of the day, was desperately cold. The walls were uninsulated and had half-inch cracks running up and down; a bitter wind routinely swept into the barn like icy, frost-covered Arctic demons. At night I was cold in my bed and I wondered what it was like for Shh who had no protection other than his hair which had begun to grow longer.

A foreshadowing of things to come first struck me when Shh whimpered whenever I blew my warm breath onto his half-frozen nose. Something hurt him. He used to get up to greet me whenever I entered the chicken barn, but now he stayed on his straw bed as though he didn't care whether I was there or not. Even bones from the butcher wouldn't rouse him. After a while Shh began to drag his legs as though they were a pair of dead limbs along for the ride. At school I checked the encyclopedia under "dog diseases" and discovered that Shh had developed a deadly disease called degenerative myelopathy. I quickly grew desperate – scared enough to pray to God to heal him. I bargained with God saying I would be kinder to my sisters if He would heal Shh.

My dog was obviously in great pain. This almost broke my heart, and sometimes I would cry into Shh's fur until he licked my salty cheeks. His whimpering bothered me the most because I believed this to be a sign of acute suffering that I could do nothing about. Finally, I prayed that he would die.

My feeling of helplessness grew until a thought, wild and wrong, came to me: I could kill Shh. The first time this occurred to me, I cried myself to sleep because the idea was so sinful. I thought of it all the next day, and when I came home from school, I decided to give up skiing in favour of lying in the straw with Shh, cradling him in my arms as if he were a baby. He dragged himself over to a piece of bread I had soaked in warm water but, after he bit at it, he heaved it up and lay whimpering, unmoving in the cold straw.

Thinking about Shh's pain made me resolute. Earlier I had shared my dilemma with a friend, and he offered to loan me his single-shot rifle. The next day, Saturday, I told Mama I was going skiing, but, instead, I hid my skis behind the chicken barn and walked the mile across town to my friend's house. I was thinking so hard about what I was about to do that I scarcely felt the bitter wind.

My friend showed me how to use his rifle and, although I had never shot a gun before, I found it pretty simple. I walked home with it, trying to look like a hunter, tall and older than my thirteen years.

I carried the rifle over my shoulder down Main Street and nobody stopped me. I took the back way through the trees and sneaked into the chicken barn.

"Shh," I called, and he raised his ears but stayed put. I leaned the gun against the wall near him and walked over to my dog and knelt beside him. "Remember when I told you how much I loved you?" I whispered, ruffling the back of his head. "With all my heart and my arms and my voice and whatever extra I could offer?" He whimpered and I remembered the encyclopedia most descriptively saying how much pain degenerative myelopathy caused. "You're not going to hurt any longer," I said and picked up the gun. I took a bullet from my pant pocket, slid it into the slot and pulled back the bolt. It was loaded. Impulsively, I laid the rifle down. "I can't do it!" I whispered. Then I remembered Jack's saying, "*Can't* is a coward's word."

Abruptly, in a great hurry, I picked up the loaded gun, aimed it between Shh's eyes, and pulled the trigger. The sound was more like a loud thud than a bang, but Shh's head dropped to the straw, his tongue hanging out of his mouth. With my toe I carefully pushed at his body. He was dead.

I pulled him onto the large piece of cardboard I had found in the school's garbage. Grabbing the cardboard with both hands, I pulled it backwards out of the chicken barn and over the slippery snow to a hollow beside the creek. Pulling my boot sideways, I pulled snow over Shh's body until it was covered. In spring the overflowing creek filled the hollow and rid it of whatever had accumulated over the winter. Shh's final grave would be wherever the rush of the spring flood took him.

I walked toward our house, trying to decide what I would tell Mama why I looked so exhausted. Whatever lie I told her, God would have to forgive me.

My Phobias

Two emotional phobias haunted me into adulthood; this double trouble ruined countless hours of my life. It seemed a hex oppressed me, although as I grew to be a man, I sometimes blamed pure Chance, that great Designer of Destinies.

I became irrationally afraid of thunderstorms the summer after my ninth birthday. In southern Manitoba, a hot summer day often ended with dark clouds on the western horizon. The most formidable clouds stretched laterally and low, south to north. They floated heavily, packed with faraway explosions of brilliance and sound. Other clouds, white and billowy, soon disappeared, as though escaping from too much passion. My fearful trembling reached from inside my body to my fingertips.

In the west, lightning streaked brilliant and thin, as though guided by a twitchy hand moving in a quick scramble of light. On this day, thunder did not reach me, and I felt a brief respite from fear, but my urge to use the outhouse soon increased. I ran to the tiny building on our yard wondering whether I could finish before the storm arrived or be caught with my pants down. I laughed nervously at my pun.

Once I was inside the outhouse, a volley of raindrops pounded briefly on the tin roof like a burst of furious words. Belligerent thunder echoed. Hunched over, eyes squeezed shut to keep the next lightning flash away, I prayed desperately for the storm to stop. God seemed deaf or, worse still, God didn't much care.

Clouds soon edged around the town's northern circumference, and I got up and ran to our house. The storm's intensity had passed, but as I ran to our home, I wondered whether a freak bolt would strike me dead. I raced as though finishing a sprint in the Manitoba Provincial Track and Field finals.

The dreadful anxiety which surfaced whenever portents of a summer storm appeared was paired with a second phobia: I was desperately afraid of dogs. My spine tingled if I even saw a picture of a dog. Quiet ones were the most intimidating. Silent, staring ones made terror my master. No town regulations held owners responsible for their dogs, so I especially dreaded walking beside hedges fronting houses where dogs might lie. I knew that most dogs romped happily with little children, but such a rational thought made no impression on my fear. I shared my phobias with no one because shame kept me silent with my brother, Jack, and I didn't want to worry Mama.

The second year that Jack was away from home in summer, a night storm blew in. I had a room to myself, Papa was working the bakery night shift, and Mama slept in the bedroom across from me. The storm seemed far away, but I hid under the covers because even mild storms caused me dreadful fear, and the blankets diminished lightning streaks. After a minute of silence, I let my guard down and pulled the covers down.

A huge rumble of thunder rolled over the house, and I jumped up and ran to Mama's room.

"What's wrong?" she asked, blinking awake. I stood speechless, trying to hide my trembling. Mama leaned on an elbow and rubbed her eyes. "It's all right," she said, and threw her cover aside to make room for me. "The storm's leaving, but there's room in here for both of us."

I was twelve years old and embarrassed, but my terror felt like something alive in my stomach. I jumped onto the big bed and pulled the cover over me. I lay beside her, tense as wire, with my back turned to her and my eyes pinched shut. She said, "Go to sleep, Henry. The storm's nearly over." She stroked my forehead with her fingers. Our bare feet touched, and I jumped.

The next morning, I woke up alone in Mama's bed and looked through the window. There were no clouds, and the sky was blue. I whispered a prayer of thanks to Jesus.

The library in Morden had one row of encyclopedias and I read everything I could find about lightning. One volume explained why thunder sounded after lightning: the two happen at the same time, but light, travelling so much faster, arrives first, so thunder seems to happen later. Light moves 186,222 miles per second, said the thick book. Per second? Really? The earth's equator was 25,000 miles around. This meant light could travel around the earth more than seven times in one second. I felt glad that mental arithmetic came easily to me but petrified by the power of light.

Sound travelled much more slowly: 742 miles per hour, or 343 metres per second. If thunder crashed a second after the lightning lit up my room, the lightning strike was less than three football fields away. That seemed close. Eventually I calculated how long it would take for thunder to reach me by counting the seconds after a bolt because I liked science and this information might make me less fearful. But my fear of the phenomenon itself was my prime reason for checking it out, not any interest in science.

The encyclopedia also said the fear aroused by any phobia is greatly out of proportion to what is warranted. I understood this, but what I grasped with my brain refused to affect my emotional response to thunderstorms and to dogs.

I read that such undue fear may be picked up by emulating someone who already has the phobia. I remember when I was little and a severe thunderstorm developed overnight, Mama roused and gathered us in the pantry, a small room without windows. Our frightened Mama told us we were safer here if a lightning bolt hit our house. Should a fire develop, she said, we could all run out of the house together. Although lightning never struck our house, Mama kept gathering us whenever a thunderstorm woke her at night. I learned my fear of lightning from Mama.

One night, after midnight, when everyone but Kay and Pete and Papa was at home sleeping, thunder woke her up, and Mama summoned us to the windowless pantry. We seven sat on the pantry floor anticipating the thunderstorm would worsen. It did. The light and sound came simultaneously. Every corner in the little room lit up. The strike's sound was like a powerful "Crack!" and the thunder's echoes were quick, brief, and exceedingly loud. We all jumped, and someone gave a sharp intake of breath. My mouth was dry. I was on the floor squeezing Martha's hand and I leaned into the warmth of her body. "Did that one hit the house?" I whispered.

"Hope not," she said, and giggled nervously. No smell of smoke followed. The storm soon moved away, and we all hurried back to bed. I fell asleep quickly, relieved by the abrupt end of this particular *Blitzkrieg*.

The next morning Jack called from outside the house and beckoned. I caught up with him when he said, "Look," and pointed to the yard's biggest ash tree split down its trunk. The sickly whiteness of its core reminded me of the time I last saw a pig slaughtered. Tree flesh, I thought, and felt my stomach turn. Lightning had ripped the tree open in a long gash and half of one side stood erect while the other clung to the original trunk; the crown lay in the water. Like a million spark plugs going off at the same instant, a fiery axe head had plunged through the pouring rain and struck a horrific blow. Already leaves were beginning to whither, and soon the tree would die.

"I hope it never hits the house," I said, scared all over again.

"Who knows?" said Jack. "Who knows?"

A Big Truck

Status issues unrelated to income sometimes made life extra interesting. Billy's father, Mr. Friesen to me, drove a big truck used for hauling bentonite from a mine nearby. Sometimes he brought the huge truck home for the weekend and we boys in the West End thought this was super special. All of us found time on either Saturday or Sunday to check it out.

We took turns sitting inside the truck, pretending to drive. The younger boys made sounds like R R R R r-r-r-r-r-R-R-R-r-r-! The bigger boys pretended to shift gears driving up a steep hill, and Billy got loads of social credit for having a father who not only drove a truck for a living but was allowed to drive it home on weekends. Billy and his brothers were totally popular via this new credit-by-association. I envied them.

Billy's father had little schooling compared to Papa who had legitimate accountancy training from a Russian school, and while he applied to many businesses in Morden, he was routinely refused work. To his total surprise and great disappointment, he discovered that a good quality job would be unavailable to him in Canada. Billy's father's job had no more quality status than Papa's, but it was more secure. It would probably outlive him. I wondered why Papa did not drive a truck for a living. It would be so much easier than the way he now worked, so frightfully hard. Could this actually happen? What a great idea! I would have to ask Jack about that.

Boyfriends and Kisses

My sister Helen loved and married steady Menno Braun, but that happened only after she'd given up other boyfriends. She fell for Jake, a redheaded guy, in her late teens. He loved to laugh and exercised this characteristic far more than most people. I was thirteen and beginning to lose, very slowly, a certain innocence.

I enjoyed making Jake's self-confidence melt, but he had a car I wanted a ride in, and I knew he'd have to like me before that would happen. I tried different approaches. Mostly they were nice things like, "Have another cookie," or a slap on the back and saying in as low a voice as I could muster, "How's it going, Buddy?" This approach didn't work, so I decided humour might do the trick.

One early evening the two of us sat in our living room waiting for Helen to finish her makeup. I asked him, "Hey, Jake, how do you manage to kiss Helen when you're laughing all the time? Those must be short kisses, eh?" I knew I shouldn't talk so brazenly to my sister's boyfriend, and I had given my opening question a lot of thought. I couldn't come up with anything except that kissing and laughing at the same time must be physically impossible. I enjoyed being a smartass.

Jake's face turned red, and I could tell he had to think hard of the right thing to say. He laughed, finally, just as Helen came into the room. She looked at Jake's red face and glared at me. "Hank, have you been minding your manners?"

I said, "If manners were so important, I'd have been born with them," and I laughed at my cleverness. They didn't think my little joke was funny.

Helen said, "Hank, you're the limit. C'mon, Jake, let's go." Jake jumped up, and they left the room before I could embarrass them further.

Maybe, I thought, I shouldn't be such a wiseacre when this guy could, potentially, join our family. Truthfully, being alone with adults actually made me nervous. I used humour to cover my fear of looking stupid. I'd rather be a court jester than a fool. Sometimes I was both. I heard the car leave with an adolescent roar.

At 10:30 Helen and Jake drove up our driveway very quietly, lights out. They didn't come in. Fifteen minutes later Mama said to me from where she was knitting some wool socks, "What are they doing out there so long? They must be getting cold." So wise about many things, and fifty-four years old, Mama couldn't figure out why two young people would spend time sitting in a car, in the dark.

"They're talking, Mama," I said, "and besides, they've got the motor running and the heater will be on." I tried to calm her because I was afraid she'd go out and investigate. I added, "I think they want to be private."

"Don't be silly," she said. "Anyway, it's way past your bedtime. Scoot."

The Pileated Woodpecker

Papa borrowed a hand scythe from a friend, and Jack taught me how to use it. I was trying, by myself, to cut the grass between the north side of our house and the Canadian Pacific Railway property, when I heard a woodpecker's peck-peck-pecking on a tree. At thirteen, I was soon bored with my job, and I leaned the scythe against the maple tree and looked for the bird. The sound had come from above, so that's where I looked – and that's where a large pileated wood-pecker clung to the side of a tree, pecking.

It turned its huge head the better part of a half-circle. At school I had seen pictures, but never in real life had I run across a live pileated woodpecker. As big as a large crow, it started pecking again.

I sat motionless. The bird resumed its pecking so efficiently that soon half its body disappeared into the hole it was making. It worked like a machine. How could a bird peck so hard without hurting its brain? I decided that the next day I'd do what Jack would do and read about it in the library. From the screen door Emma called, and I knew Mama had a chore for me. After I had taken out the ashes from the bake oven, I ran back to the tree. The woodpecker was gone, so I clambered up the maple, sweeping away the remaining chips from the branches as I climbed.

I reached into the hole. With my fingertips I felt something soft and feathery. It couldn't be! I reached deeper, got a better grip on the softness and pulled out a pileated woodpecker. It never moved even the slightest. For an instant I thought it must be stuffed.

Holding the woodpecker carefully with one hand, I climbed down, placing my feet on the dead branches near the trunk, more afraid that I would drop the bird than that I would fall. I carefully sat down on the ground and looked at what I had in my hand.

The woodpecker's beak was as long as its head, and the streaks around its neck reminded me of a baby zebra's hide. Its head was tufted with a red crest brighter than barn paint. I held the bird with one hand and stroked its back with the other. The downy softness reminded me of baby skin. Marble eyes stared at me, and I couldn't decide whether I should let it go for its own sake or keep its beauty for myself.

A hair-raising sense of wonder filled me, and in my gut a tingling stirred. I felt certain this had something to do with noticing God, just as I had felt something sacred when lying under the pines, or when the wind slipped past my cheeks skiing down Baldy Hill.

The flashy woodpecker was so untamed and so wild that something inside me said I should let it go. Totally unique, utterly itself, it needed to be shared. The huge bird and I locked eyes.

Suddenly I stood up and shouted, "I'll share it with everybody!" and I threw it underhanded and with both hands high into the air. At its apex, the woodpecker remained, for an instant, as taut as when I held it. Then the bird unbound its wings, defied gravity, and flapped away.

Letter to Jack

Well, have you had enough yet of riding the train across Canada? It must be fun to be a porter. I'd like to do that someday.

Yesterday I caught a bird. A pileated woodpecker, the biggest kind, about like a crow. I just reached into a hole in the dry maple by our bedroom window and grabbed the feathers and pulled it out. What a thrill! After a while I had to let it go because I thought it might die, it was so still. While

I had it in my hand, I thought how you said God is in nature.
I sort of understand what you mean.
  It was beautiful with a huge yellow beak.
  Your brother,
  Hank
  P.S. Don't fall off the train (ha ha). When are you
  coming home.

Dead Horse Creek

Dead Horse Creek's ugly name hardly reflected the affection I felt for it. Meandering fifty metres from our house, the creek delineated the west side of our property from the town's. In summer I swam in the creek with the other boys, in winter it was my private skating rink, in fall it barely trickled and I avoided it, and in spring I watched the exciting flash flood which Mama hated, because it annually filled our house with a foot of dirty water. Every season the water rose and fell like some teachers' moods. I never tired of watching its predictable display.

During winter, the wind and the snow and the thermometer determined how often I used the ice. If the frost came hard and quickly, the creek was glossy-smooth, and I skated for hours. If snow fell during an early frost, the ice surface was bumpy. A blizzard guaranteed great drifts that made it impossible to skate except for a few long stretches of wind-swept ice, as unwrinkled as that of the Morden Curling Rink.

In early springtime, I mostly watched. The snow-covered surface turned to cold, flowing water. I loved the creek for some of the same reasons I loved trees: in their seasonal changes each altered its particular beauty. The creek, mostly white from its snow covering, changed to black patches of ice reflecting the black shades of water below and, once the spillway overflowed, the contrast between the foaming, light grey water and the dark, leafless bushes alongside the creek created an otherworldliness I would always remember. Spring changed the sounds that came from the creek. Summer birds that sang sweetly weren't back yet, and in their place the sound of breaking ice together with the everlasting chirping of the noisy sparrows broke through the bitterly cold air.

Swimming with Billy

Where the flooding creek turned sharply north, the fast water had, over decades, intruded deeply into the high bank facing west, and each year the flooding gouged out more and more chunks of dirt. A natural swimming hole developed. In summer, my friends and I spent hours jumping from the high bank into seven feet of water. We swam and shouted and dived and played water games. Sometimes Bill and I irritated each other.

One day I executed a steep dive from the top of the bank straight to the bottom, "You're stirring up the mud!" shouted Bill when I surfaced near him. "Don't dive to the bottom like that!" He turned his behind skyward and slid smoothly, headfirst down and away from me.

It was true that our pool was less clear now than before my dive, but whose pool was this anyway? "Baloney!" I hollered when he came up. "The deeper I can dive, the better I like it," and I slapped my hand flat on the water toward him, spraying his face.

"How can you be so stupid?" he shouted. He was getting riled up.

"You're lots stupider than I am," I hollered back. We were getting mad at each other. Head down, bum-up, I dived again.

The contrast between our stupid argument and the peaceful feel of the water calmed me. More than anything I loved the water's smoothness when I swam under its surface. Nothing could reach me, touch me, tell me where I should go, or what I should be doing. I prized the isolation, the disengagement from noise, the voluntary exile. I felt safe. My extended body slipped easily through the sweep of water flowing past me like billowing clouds. I was only sorry that I had to surface to breathe.

When I emerged, Billy had gone home. My serenity disappeared. I felt sorry about our disagreement. I really liked Bill more than I sometimes let on. In fact, he was my best friend. I would have to make up with him.

The Beavers

The evening light from May through August proved an asset when hiding from the beavers as I watched them. Last fall, they had built a house of branches and mud not far from our house. Jack said they swam into their house near the bottom of the creek through a small hole they made. Summer days, he said, they swam through this opening, and slept during the day. I thought of it as a safe house, and watched, entranced. Mama, who considered me fidgety (rather like Papa), never knew how long I could sit on the grassy bank as still as a Buddhist.

One evening, a beaver swam past me, its humped back and webbed feet visible just under the clear water. The beaver climbed onto its house and began chewing the green twigs it had dragged there. I focussed on its whiskers, its nostrils and its eyes. Totally absorbed, I marvelled at the beaver's glossy fur gleaming a few feet away from me. Farther down the creek a dead branch must have fallen, and I heard a second beaver's tail whack the water, hard. Hiding noiselessly, I felt as though I were in the middle of a crime novel in a story about beavers sneaking around, swimming away from danger that might strike at any time. For a minute, I was almost scared.

Flight, Jack once told me, was a beaver's only protection from predators. I didn't understand which category tail-slaps fell into, but this instinct to warn fascinated me. I would have to stay after school to study it further, in the library.

In the silence between tail slaps I recalled lying on Baldy Hill with the hard snow under my body. I was too young to understand what "God" might be, but I could grasp, somewhat, the word "sacred." This word always prompted me to think about Dead Horse Creek and skiing at Baldy Hill, and, lately, "The Island." I wondered why I had this feeling of someone else being there every time I was alone in one of these three places. What Preacher Friesen called "holy" rose in my mind. Maybe the words "nature" and "holy" and "sacred" were actually names for God. Recently I had wondered whether the word "sacred" was a synonym for "nature." Each of these words appealed to me, and for the first time I noticed how strangely organized the world was.

Skiing

The Pembina Valley, a series of hills and valleys running a mile southwest of Morden, edged around my hometown. Any hill was in striking contrast to the thousands of square miles of flat prairie farmland that lay around us. An immense amount of grain could easily be harvested annually and exported to the world because the prairie, "breadbasket of the world," lay as level as a pancake. I loved the panoramic prairie, the fields of grain and the horizon unfolding in every direction. An exception to all this openness were the hills of the Pembina Valley.

For each of the winter school days from age eleven to fourteen, I rushed home where I strapped my rubber buckle overshoes onto my wooden skis and coasted off our yard. Because we lived on the west end of town, I headed directly to the flat countryside. Ski poles pushing into the snow, I slid across the winter emptiness of open fields where a mile away Baldy Hill, the first rise of the Pembina Valley, waited for me. More than anywhere else, that is where I wanted to be.

Trying to stay in shape, I gave myself amateur skiing lessons. I skied as fast as I could in the softest snow I could find. When I approached breathlessness, I looked for packed snow where I could effortlessly skim over the hard top until I had my breath back. I repeated this until I reached the hills.

From the bottom of Baldy Hill, I zigzagged my way up, then skied down in an exhilarating rush, then climbed back up again, then swooped down. I did this in an ad hoc fashion until I was tired. When I reached the top the last time for that day, I poled my way to a clump of pine trees where I unsnapped my overshoes and lay down on my back on top of the snow. Under the shadow of the pines, this bank of solid snow became my frost-hardened bed.

I was alone. The winter sun touched the northwest horizon, and a February half-moon rose in the east as though cooperating. The crystalized bed of snow easily tolerated my weight, and I closed my eyes. After a while, silence and time slowed my heartbeat. Every day I whispered, "Are you here, God?" and then I listened. The quietness deepened, and a particular peacefulness slipped, as though on silent skis, toward me where I lay on my back underneath the pines. No breeze moved, and the cold gentleness reminded me of quiet, calm night-skating on Dead Horse Creek. Gone was the fearful threat of summer lightning. The snow, the moon, and my boy's body melded. I was content.

I called what was happening "Talking to God." In our overlapping conversation, I listened more than I spoke. I relaxed, not toward sleep, but toward an awareness of each sensation nature evoked. God was here — if not the God of my church, then at least a boy's consciousness of something special. My physical environment merged with the numinous, and the cold night scarcely chilled me. Too much was happening.

Spring Flash Floods

Centuries before heavy equipment arrived to build the Morden Dam, the Dead Horse Creek functioned as an outlet for enormous wetlands which began the way lowland waters are born: after a heavy rain, rivulets of water crawled out of the earth and formed huge puddles which joined even bigger puddles. Vegetation grew, more rain fell. Small streams and larger rivulets flowed down from higher ground, more vegetation sprang and over multiple centuries, the annual cycle created a swamp. Each spring the rains caused excess water to gather at the swamp's lowest point. Over time, a small creek formed and led the water away.

Lake Minnewasta was sometimes more than useful. In 1951, because the small town of Morden needed more water, engineers built a dam and a spillway on the east side of the swamp. In April, temperatures rose quickly and often the melting snow filled the new lake beyond the dam's capacity. The only exit was the spillway, a huge width of concrete at one end of the dam which acted as an open valve allowing the water to pour over. When the spring melt came suddenly, an eighteen-inch wall of water thundered over the spillway with a noise that kept timid people away. At the spillway's bottom, the creek formed.

My friends and I hitchhiked the two-mile gravel road from Morden whenever we could to marvel at the enormous rush of water gouging out a watery path toward Morden. The great spillway wash swept over the lowest levels of land, and the creek expanded with drama and force. Ice, sludge and melted water thrashed and sprang high, forming a quick current that circled in repeating rotations of ice-cold water. Beside the creek, branches from chokecherry bushes broke, and pieces of ice jammed in against the creek's banks.

As though in a race, the surge struck Morden's West End where it burst and spread into a flash flood. Low-lying gardens disappeared under water. The sun had long ago set, and streetlights shone yellow; their light struck the water and reflected back into the night sky. In the West End, whole sections of roads succumbed as the flood fled around the centre of town.

At home, my siblings piled the best furniture onto the oldest. They hoisted the couch onto four wooden chairs. No electricity meant no dealing with refrigerators and powered stoves, but the earthen cellar filled, and mud and water pushed up through the kitchen's trap door in the floor. When I got home from watching the creek rise, a foot of water covered the downstairs floor of our house, and light from the kerosene lamps shone back from the dirty water.

It abated the next morning, leaving a layer of slime and mud on every square foot of living space on our ground floor. The water drained slowly, giving Mama time to consider how she would clean up the horrible mess. A garden hoe and a shovel were good for getting rid of the mud, but could she return the cheap linoleum to its usual shine?

Her insistence on cleanliness led Mama to wonder how long it would take for the muddy water to disappear from the cellar. Might someone lend Jack a pump? With the water gone, she and the girls would wash and replace the shelves she had stored in the chicken barn a day ago. They would replace the glass quarts of canned cucumbers and fruit now standing on the dining room table. Mama's unstoppable determination surfaced, and she thought: the cellar might be a hole under the house, but she would make it a clean hole.

The F-word

One summer evening, before the sun was fully gone, Jack and I walked west along the railroad tracks near our house. A mile behind us, smoke pouring from its steel smokestack, a freight train pulled out of Morden's station, whistled its way toward the West End, accelerated past Jack and me, and headed for the faraway curve. After the caboose clattered past, I stepped back onto the iron rail, tried to balance, slipped, and dropped six inches onto the wooden railway ties.

"What's this?" I asked, picking up a strange-looking disc the size of a quarter.

Jack smiled. "I put a penny on the track before the train got here. A hundred train wheels just drove over it." I examined the flattened disc more carefully and, sure enough, the face of King George VI looked like a stretched clown's head.

Jack was seven years older than I, and very smart. He was my brother and I believed him when he told me things. Today I asked him how come our sisters never used the f-word. Recently I had learned how babies were made, and still felt embarrassed. I wouldn't say the f-word either, but I felt like making a joke. Should I? Yeah, why not.

I said, "I guess the girls think that they'll get pregnant with the devil's baby if they say the f-word." I laughed.

Jack didn't even smile. "Hank, get serious," he said. "Two of the girls are going through the boy-crazy stage right now. They don't think much. At least not about this. Right now, they believe in the evil power of certain words they think are bad, and they won't use them. That's a superstition people used to believe and practise a lot."

"Why don't people do that now?"

"They do. Look at the girls. That's exactly what we're talking about."

"You mean," I said, "the girls believe some words have actual power?"

"Sure seems like it," Jack said. "That's not new. In medieval times people got killed for using particular words. I read about it in a book. Nowadays, self-righteous people still avoid certain words. Like good Christians, they never use swear words. Psychologists say they're practising magical thinking."

"Magical thinking?"

"Yes, magical thinking." We heard the train's faint *w - h - o - o - o o o o o* at a distant crossing.

"Really?"

"Really." Jack knew almost everything, so I believed him, but I still wish he had laughed at my joke about babies and the devil.

Boobie: The Great Knockout

We never thought of Boobie Bergen as a regular friend, but today he joined Alvin and Billy and me walking home from school. Other than Boobie, we were all thirteen, and thought Boobie peculiar and immature for fourteen. We three gave him lots of latitude, though, thinking his ill father was at the root of his personality, his abrupt movements from exaggerated noisiness to sullen silence.

Alvin was chewing on an apple he had kept from lunch. Billy and I were taking turns kicking an empty Pork 'n Beans can down the road. A car blew its horn behind us, and we moved to the side of the road.

The wind blew easily. It was a fine and sunny day. Earlier, the weather was cold, and clouds were thick. Now we stuffed our toques into our oversized parka pockets and pulled down our zippers. Winter boots, intended for this morning's temperature, felt heavy. We unbuckled them and dragged our shoes through the snow. Winter underwear was an insult to the day.

Boobie suddenly shouted, "Holy Roller, you!" and threw a hunk of broken snow. It hit Billy's shoulder.

Billy had a super loud voice. He shouted back, "Shut your mouth! Or I'll shut it for you!" and then he added, "Boobie Baby." We all thought Boobie's name was a joke, but nobody ever referred to it so directly, or so negatively. Trouble brewed.

Alvin turned off in front his house. "So long," he said. Billy and I waved.

Alvin looked over his shoulder in time to hear Boobie say, "Hey, Billy, you must pay your janitor a lot, so he'll keep the floor clean for all you Holy Rollers!"

Billy was angry but he spoke quietly. "I'll tell you once more, shut your chicken-shit mouth!" and he approached Boobie and blocked his way.

From his yard, Alvin called, "Hey, you guys, take it easy," and came back to where we had stopped. A truck in low gear, carrying sand, passed us but nobody waved.

Boobie said, "All that speaking in tongues must make you clean your mouth more than most people do, eh?" He tried to give Billy a shove but Billy, quick on his feet, moved in on Boobie and swung his fist once. Luck or skill, he hit Boobie directly on his chin knocking his head back. He fell to the ground like a heavy stone dropping through water. Nobody moved or said anything.

Then I called, "You knocked him out, Billy!" I felt victorious, as though I claimed the right to a school cheerleaders' triumph, but Billy went through a transformation. He was beside himself with anxiety.

"I'm sorry!" he shouted, stricken. "I killed you!" and he fell to his knees beside the unconscious Boobie. "I'm sorry, I'm sorry!" he shouted. "Don't die! Please don't die!" and he grabbed some snow and rubbed it on Boobie's face and put his mouth beside his ear. "Forgive me!"

Boobie opened his eyes. Alvin helped him sit up.

"What happened?" Boobie mumbled.

"I hit you," said Billy. "I thought you were dead!"

Boobie got up. His white face and his bare head shook a little. He felt his jaw and looked at his fingers for blood. There was none. He took a deep breath and spat into the snow. "You stupid Pentecostal," he said.

We broke up. Alvin turned toward his home, and Billy and I headed for the railway tracks. Boobie stood alone in the snow.

The Non-Fight

During the Second World War, conscientious objectors who wished to avoid spending time in the military service were allowed to work for Alternative Services, a government organization. Mennonite pacifists were allowed to choose ministrations such as hospital work or road construction rather than join the armed forces. My older siblings chose hospital work, and registered for the Mental Health Centre in Brandon, Manitoba.

Bert Stobbe, a Grade Ten student in my class at Morden Collegiate in 1954, had non-church-going Mennonite parents who very publicly opposed any alternatives for conscientious objectors. Although the Second World War had ended years ago, people who shared the Stobbes' opinions harboured strong resentment against all pacifists who had contributed to their country only in non-violent ways. I felt strongly in favour of my church's pacifist position, while Bert shared his parents' stance. After school one day, he and I happened to meet on the school grounds.

"Hey, you bloody pacifist!" Bert shouted in my face. "Wanna fight?" He kicked me hard in the shins. It hurt a lot, but Jack had told me that sometimes it took more courage to resist fighting than to fight. I walked away. Bert ran after me and kicked me hard on my tailbone; it sizzled all the way up my spine. I turned to face him.

"You chickenshit!" he shouted. A small crowd gathered. "C'mon, take a swing at me." He stuck out his chin. Bert was taller than I was, but skinny as a post. I felt a strong urge to hit him in the face.

"I don't fight for no reason," I said.

Someone in the group hollered, "Fight! Fight! you sissy, fight!" Bert slapped at my face. I ducked and he missed, and he swung his fist, and this time he hit me squarely on my nose. I staggered back but kept my arms down.

"Baby!" someone hollered.

"Coward!"

The small crowd jeered louder, and I kept thinking how much I would like to beat up this tall weakling and have the crowd boo him instead of me. It was horribly embarrassing at fourteen to stand there and let Bert slap me around. But I believed in demonstrating my Christian beliefs rather than talking about them, so I refused to hit him back. I kept wanting to cry. Bert struck me repeatedly and I finally fell to the ground. The high schoolers drifted away. Bert gave me a hard kick in the ribs and ran after them.

I stumbled to my feet and headed home. By the time I reached the town pump, my nose had stopped bleeding and I washed the dry blood from my face. Half a thought formed in my mind as I walked the rest of the way home. I didn't like what I was thinking, so I ignored it until later.

Mama was at the far end of the garden, and I slipped unnoticed into the house. No one was home, and through the open window facing the garden I shouted, "I'm home, Mama. I'm doing homework in my room."

My voice almost broke, but Mama hollered back, "OK." I climbed the stairs to the room I had shared with Jack. I sat down and laid my arms on the table I used as my desk and put my head down. Papa was sleeping, and Emma was at a girlfriend's house. No one else lived at home anymore.

Boy, was I tired. Preacher Friesen would say "weary," and I would agree. I rested for a bit, and suddenly I began to cry. I cried hard for a long time.

When I heard Mama bang the screen door, I quickly got up, took a hanky from my pocket, and wiped my eyes until I felt I looked pretty normal. I looked into the small mirror on the wall and wiped my face some more.

At the table, Mama looked at me quizzically and I told her I'd tripped on a broken piece of wooden sidewalk and it jumped up and hit my head. There must be different kinds of lies because this one didn't bother me. Mama gave me another look but didn't say anything. I got through supper without any questions being asked. We ate without speaking.

Back in my room I finished my homework and went to bed early. I always knelt on the floor to pray before lying down, but today I flung the covers back and crawled in. I lay on my back, and the half-thought I'd had earlier began to develop.

How had my pacifistic actions helped anybody? I knew that Jesus said to turn the other cheek, but whom had that helped today? Not Bert: he would revel in his meanness. Not the jeering crowd; they had been entertained. It did nothing for me except make me feel humiliated and scared for the next day. Maybe, I thought, we didn't understand what Jesus really meant, and I should have slugged Bert. For the first time in my life, what the Bible said didn't make sense in its usual unerring way.

This last thought made me feel so guilty, I slid out of bed and dropped to my knees. I prayed the same way I did every night.

Harvey Flett, Bully

Driven by a need to rectify justice, I overdramatized the need to see right win over wrong. I was tenacious about being "open" (what I called honest), even if I risked nasty consequences. Seeing the truth *done* was an inordinately risky characteristic of mine which did me plenty of harm. A doggedness about sticking with principles pre-occupied me into adulthood. Probably my overplayed "honesty" was learned from Papa's example. Whatever the outside source, my motivation included a childish sense of martyrdom. I maintained this characteristic for years.

Harvey Flett, a rugged boy two years older than I, disliked me. One day he said he was going to rip my ears off, and I said, "Oh, I'm so scared I'm shaking in my runners," and I put on a show of shaking with fear.

Bill was with me and half-whispered, "Stop that, Hank, he's going to kick the crap out of you."

"So?" I said. "So?" I spoke as though an army stood behind me.

"Look," I said to Harvey who had his face in mine, "see how scared I am?" and I grinned.

Harvey swung a thick arm at me, palm open so he could later say he only slapped me, but he used the calloused heel of his hand, and struck me under my left eye. I registered the pain and felt the swelling, but I stood as tall as I could manage. He wandered off, yelling and swearing at me over his shoulder.

"I told you," Billy said. "That guy could kill you, but you mock him. What are you trying to prove?" He looked at my face. "That's a terrible welt he gave you." I ran my fingertips over the abrasion. They came back with blood, and I felt a big bulge on my cheekbone.

"I don't care if he does it again," I said, squinting at Billy with my functioning eye.

"Are you nuts?" exclaimed Billy. "Do you want to die? What's the matter with you?"

All the way home I asked myself this question: Was something wrong with me? Did I actually want to die? No way, I said half aloud, that's stupid. I simply couldn't tolerate bullies, and enjoyed mocking them more than anything else, even if it got me a bruised face. I wasn't entirely free of my own bullying, so it would seem I owned my anger. This made me worse than a hapless victim.

Abusing Ronny Derksen

Ronny Derksen lived two blocks from us, on the other side of Dead Horse Creek. Even for Grade Seven he was a small guy; he delivered the *Winnipeg Tribune* to West End customers.

Partly, I didn't like Ronny Derksen because his family didn't go to a Mennonite church. They didn't go to any church at all, actually, and my fourteen-year-old brain, so over-committed to my own church, thought he had no right to a Mennonite family name. I told this to Jack, and he said, "Don't be ridiculous." I clung to my opinion, and Jack didn't say anything more about it.

I knew I shouldn't hate anyone, but I hated Ronny's face. Whenever I saw him, I said, "Hey, Turkey-Durkey, you jerk, what did you steal today?" or "How come you walk so slow, you lazy Durkey?" or "Nobody likes your ugly mug, you Turkey-Durkey!"

I was two years older than Ronny, and he was scared of me, a nice change from my being frightened of so many other guys. He brought the worst out in me. I had never bullied anybody in my life, but I always wanted to beat him up, the Mennonite traitor. Whenever he saw me, he put his head down and kept on walking.

One day after school, a spring wind dragged rain clouds across Morden. Ronny came walking toward me and, as we passed, I leaned a shoulder into him and gave him a heavy bodycheck. He lurched sideways, and his *Winnipeg Tribune* canvas bag slipped from his shoulder. A gust of wind yanked a paper out and blew it down the street.

When Ronny got up, I stood between him and his bag. "So sorry," I said, and looked around to see if anyone was watching. "Here, let me help you with a few more," I said and grabbed some papers out of his bag and, with both hands, threw them, underhanded, high into the air. They flew wildly apart, and I laughed.

"See that?" I shouted. "Think you could do that?"

He scrambled to his feet, and I noticed tears sliding down his cheeks. This infuriated me. "You traitor!" I hollered, and swung my arm to slap his face, but he ducked and grabbed his bag and ran. At the street corner where he lived, he turned, and I yelled as loudly as I could, "You little chicken shit!"

Sudden hard rain struck my face, and I hurried home.

Mama and Papa and I had supper. We ate quietly until there was a knock on the door. Papa called, "Come in," and Ronny's father pushed the outside door open. My heart jumped.

"Mr. Neufeld," Mr. Derksen said, "Could you come outside for a minute?" Papa nodded, got up, and the two fathers banged the screen door behind them.

Mama's and my eyes met, and it came to me for the first time that I had done something much more than tease Ronny. I, more than anybody, should have remembered the deep-down fear that bullying causes. I had betrayed the pacifist peace of my personal beliefs.

Papa came back in, sat down and resumed eating. I couldn't swallow my food. When Papa finished eating, Mama cleared the dishes from the table. Papa spoke quietly. "Mr. Derksen says you've been tormenting his son." He took a red handkerchief from his pocket and wiped his mouth. "Is this true?"

I felt an urge to go to the outhouse, as if I could see a row of thunderclouds developing on the horizon. I looked at Papa out of the corner of my eye. "Yes," I said.

"Why?" Papa didn't seem angry.

I told the truth. "I don't like him," I said.

"You're fourteen years old and know better than to hurt people because you dislike them," said Papa. "You certainly haven't learned that in *this* house." He raised his voice. "Have you?"

I said, "No," but my voice broke. I was sure a beating would be next, except that Papa spoke so deliberately and calmly.

From the sink, Mama clattered the dishes, then turned toward us, needing to hear how this conversation would end.

Papa said, "I told Mr. Derksen that such behaviour would cease." He stood up. "Today." Although he was not a tall man, he loomed over me. "Was I right?"

Papa had never had a civil conversation with me about my behaviour, and I wondered why he was hesitant to beat me.

I said, "Yes," and he sat down.

"Go now," Papa said, "And pay him a dollar for his lost papers." He reached for the German *Rundschau* and unfolded it.

"I can go?" I asked, bewildered. Papa tilted his head toward the screen door. I scraped my chair back and hurried out of the house. I looked toward "The Island," paused a second, then turned and ran to the outhouse.

Choir Practice

Alvin Reimer, my good church friend, came from a musical family that formed a band. Alvin played first violin, another brother played second, a third brother stood over six feet tall as he bowed the big bass, and the oldest played piano. Their father stroked the cello. The four boys and one sister came from a home where Mom and Dad were strictly in charge about pretty well everything their children did. My own mama and papa were permissive about my general whereabouts, except for mealtime, when you either showed up or excused yourself earlier.

Alvin and I walked or biked the mile to school together. When he turned sixteen, he occasionally drove his father's half-ton truck. Being friends with Alvin meant I didn't walk all the way to school very often. Being on good terms with him meant a whole lot of other things: arriving at school in the truck gave me status and, if I was lucky, it gave me a girl to squeeze between the two of us. On days when Alvin wanted the girl to himself, I walked.

Because singing was such an important part of our church life, we joined the adult choir when we turned sixteen. This meant that every Friday night we were assigned to choir practice; we were not allowed to skip. Not that we would have wanted to. We were beginning the initial turn toward maleness and a main part of getting older meant paying minute attention to all the girls and women sitting in front of us. We were the only boys in this initiation and arrived at important conclusions by ourselves. We hinted a lot, but never talked privately to each other about "the real thing."

Alvin and I joined at the same time. He sang bass and I sang tenor, and consequently we were assigned different places to sit. This didn't prevent us from communicating, however, because he sat directly behind me. Passing notes proved as workable as in English class. And more fun.

We developed a fine system of communicating with hand and body movements. If one of us stroked his chin (where faint hopes of a beard already grew), and if this gesture was accompanied with a quick sideways jerk of one's head in the direction of a particular girl, it meant, "Boy, I'd like to spend some time alone with her!" If this was followed with a fit of coughing, the message changed to my long request, "Can you get the truck tomorrow, and can I use it? I'll get her to come with me during physics class. OK?" This message to Alvin was always answered with the crash of the heaviest hymn book the choir owned as he dropped it onto the hardwood floor. Everybody jumped, and Alvin quickly manufactured that look of innocence only a boy's guilt can produce. The book-dropping was a blunt return message: "Are you dreaming!?" We never dared to engage in this particular communication more than once an evening, but devised additional messages in the men's washroom, some so explicit we didn't look at each other when we practised them.

Our gesturing game proved to be so exciting, we could hardly wait for Sunday mornings when many people faced us and we could choose our own favourite woman to concentrate on and signal to each other. Much of the excitement lay in the fact that we did this in a public church service, and no one knew what we wholesome-looking boys were up to. We never missed choir practice or Sunday worship service for fifty Sundays in a row.

Toward the end of this year, Alvin and I learned more about the serious aspects of churchgoing. We grew up a little. In order to give some balance to our nonsense, we both decided to regularly practise daily devotions. Our derring-dos faded away and each of us, rather abruptly, spent time alone daily, reading the Bible and praying. Jesus became my pal.

I had initiated this for myself at Red Rock Summer Bible Camp and found that these fifteen minutes gave me thoughts and feelings similar to what had so vividly arisen at what I called my spiritual triangle, The Island, Old Baldy, and Dead Horse Creek. I had no doubt God was literally present at both my personal devotions and at my self-named triad, and that I was, in fact, spiritually touched by God. I decided to become even more rigorous with my daily devotions, more disciplined about setting aside a time at least once a day for Bible reading, prayer and meditation.

As a result of faithfully practising daily devotions, I came to believe that God Himself was literally beside me, that He actually advised me, through Scripture, about life's practical decisions, and that the contradictory elements of the Bible that troubled me would someday be explained. I came to believe that God had actually organized my discovering The Island, Old Baldy, and Dead Horse Creek in order to remind me of my other triad: Father, Son, and Holy Ghost.

Dugout Baptism

Persons who wished to join the church through baptism – mostly children of Mennonite Brethren Church members in their mid-teens – were required to share their conversion experiences with the congregation. After their oral testimony was formally accepted, they were baptized and became full members of the Morden Mennonite Brethren Church.

Many Mennonite churches' form of baptism was by "sprinkling" a dash of water on the candidate's head. Mennonite Brethren churches, however, baptized by full immersion in a convenient lake or river. The Morden Mennonite Brethren Church used a church member's dugout, a large, machine-made round hole in the earth which once had provided drinking water for cattle during dry months.

Tents were provided for changing quarters. The minister walked waist deep into the water followed by the nervous baptismal candidates. One at a time he asked them to answer "Yes" if they wished to follow Jesus' example and be baptized, thereby publicly testifying to their faith in Jesus. The minister, carefully supporting the candidates' backs with his right hand, and using his other hand to tighten around the candidates' hands in front of them, tipped them over backwards until they were fully submerged, and then raised them up to their feet. This ritual was a frightening ordeal for any person unused to water in a pond, but candidates all went through with it even when trembling with physical anxiety. For teenagers, this part of the ceremony was a cinch because most of us were swimmers, and water held no fear.

The symbolic element of baptism, a celebration of quiet joy, also posed as a public commitment. Mennonite churches practised few rituals, so when one occurred, the congregation viewed the baptismal act with a stolid happiness. Each personal baptism was a permanent statement, a joyous promise. Witnesses understood the emotional mixture of the merger happening, and here and there people wept. I knew Papa was happy for me: he cried throughout both the indoor and outdoor parts of the service.

Over the last year, I had worried a lot about my church's shortcomings, but my baptismal experience generated an amazing sense of belonging that countered such doubts. I knew baptism was a profound event, but I had not expected the depth of my fervent feeling of belonging. On baptismal Sunday, the serious puzzlements I had about God and His followers were almost eliminated by the compelling connectedness I felt. What underlined this was the gratefulness I felt for the loving way Preacher Friesen had helped Papa in the past and would likely repeat in the future.

Morden Collegiate Institute Student

I began high school in the mid '50s with less confidence than expertise. I had always felt like an outsider, but beginning in Grade Eleven my abilities in sports and in public speaking were instrumental in boosting my sense of self-worth. Becoming visibly successful meant I walked with my shoulders back, and my eyes looked ahead.

One day my English teacher asked me to read aloud from *Hamlet* to my Grade Twelve class. Sitting at my desk at the back of the classroom, I read with no stage fright and unusual confidence. The students grew still and attentive, and, for the first time in my life, I realized that I could hold an audience like my father could.

Sports in a small-town school never had much of an audience to impress, but that didn't slow me down. When scrimmage was organized over the noon hour, I skipped lunch because I'd rather play than eat. What passed for football was a scrimmage line and a wild game of bloodball. We followed our own rules, had no equipment, no referee and no fear. Our exuberance was matched only by a total disregard for physical safety. Lining up on scrimmage, we smashed into each other with a careless lack of restraint. Nobody played with more abandon than I did. After a few minutes, most boys conspicuously avoided physical contact with me; between plays they stared at me as though they'd never seen me before. My need to be better than anyone else made me unafraid, and my desire to be one of the guys inspired a heedless rush into the fray. Now that I'd found a certain success, my original lack of self-esteem turned into a need to demonstrate my right to it.

In June of Grade Twelve, my class voted for their graduation valedictorian, and they chose me. For a week, I floated like a monarch butterfly that had found its wings.

On a whim, I registered for the Southern Manitoba Speech Festival. I wrote my own speech, delivered it well, worked my way up the festival ladder, and won the trophy. I'd been feeling like a butterfly earlier, now I flew a mile high.

$\mathcal{A}$GE EIGHTEEN
TO TWENTY-TWO

Toward Becoming a Teacher

After Grade Twelve, during the months of July and August 1957, I worked at a construction firm in Carman, framing houses. In the middle of August, I began to think about my immediate future, and wondered what I should be doing about it. Mentally, I reviewed my options.

Jack had invited me to go with him to teach in Twillingate, Newfoundland under the auspices of the Mennonite Central Committee. I had no formal teacher training, but teachers were in such short supply that provinces were happy to issue a teaching permit to almost any high school graduate. The idea appealed to me, but halfway through August, plans fell through because of inter-provincial complications.

Attending university hadn't been a consideration for many reasons: in 1957, only a handful of elite high school graduates attended university, and I didn't fit that category. I also had little money to pay my way, and loans were not easily available. As well,

I had no idea what area of study I might pursue. Two or three years earlier, I would have said my studies had to cover some theological aspect of preparing to "serve the Lord," but I hadn't the slightest notion how university subject options and future church work related. Living away from home during the summer hadn't lent itself to regular church attendance which, compared to my earlier intense piety, had increased the number of basic questions I had about things spiritual.

It struck me, quite suddenly, that I should register for Normal School. Four of my siblings were teachers, Normal School was cheap (they almost paid you to come), and there existed many areas of church work where teacher training could be an asset. I applied (late) but was promptly accepted. In my diary I wrote that I had *fallen* into a teaching career.

Piano, Manitoba Normal School

One evening in September of 1957, as an eighteen-year-old student at Manitoba's Normal School, I walked into its main building to explore the huge stone structure. I heard piano music and remembered that a chapel stood somewhere in the heart of the building. I opened the outside ecclesiastical doors wide, and the sound grew louder. The music rested for a few beats, and I slipped inside.

Except for the glow of an electric lamp on top of the piano at the front of the chapel, the large, sloping space of the chapel sat in darkness in front of me. I found a chair in the back row, the piano playing continued, and I sat and listened.

Music had filled my life, but this sound felt uniquely personal, as though the piano was being played for a private audience. A certain familiarity with the rhythm made me think I had heard the music before, that I understood its language. The pianist's face was in shadow and I wondered did I know the player, or was my reaction simply a strong synchronism? I listened, and listened some more. Before the piece was over, I slipped back through the heavy doors and hurried back to my room.

Seeing Betty for the First Time

"Do you know that girl who's getting out of the cab?" I asked Harry and pointed. I had been to Normal School for a week, and Harry was a new friend.

"Sure," he said. "That's Betty Tiessen. I went to school with her at Mennonite Collegiate Institute last year."

I said, "Wow, she looks great!"

"We can get closer," said Harry.

"No," I said. "Not now. I have to go back to my room for a minute. I'll catch you later." I ran to my room at the Normal School dormitory, pulled my diary out of its drawer and, under September 9, 1957, impulsively wrote: "I just saw somebody I want to meet. Her name's Betty and I have this crazy feeling something big will happen."

Like a baseball headed for a home run, I had been struck. I'd been infatuated with girls before, but never like this. I wrote, "Maybe I'll marry her." That was preposterous – I'd never even met her. But the feeling in my gut stayed throughout supper, when I bumped into Harry again. He asked, "What's with you? Where'd you go so fast?"

"Oh," I said, "Just doing important stuff."

Falling in Love

Totally absorbed in somebody other than myself, each segment of my life suddenly included Betty. I had fallen in love with a loud thump. I took her into account in everything I did. Things that I had once considered essential became optional, and my options remained untouched. Mesmerized, I never questioned my logic, only my feelings counted.

In my life, a significant number of people have been lastingly influential on my deeper thinking, while a few have profoundly affected my *Weltanschauung*. My two children, one achingly dead and one very much alive, are imprinted on my very breath. A few people continue to catch my attention with their insights. Betty, however, is still in a category by herself. When I first saw her, my emotional life went berserk. Sixty years later, when I say, "I love you," I say it with a particular tenor in my voice that is missing when I say it to others whom I love. She has stood tall as my ally for six decades, and is my greatest inspiration.

The year I fell in love with Betty I didn't walk, I floated. When she came near me, all my senses sharpened. Even my taste for food changed because she made my mouth dry. When I first held her hand, my anticipation made me feel positively undomesticated. I experienced my new life in an extravagant, half-wild way.

In June of year's end, I was given an F in a subject called "Library." I had read a pile of books, so why the F? I hadn't submitted my *Bobbsey Twins at the Seashore* report. A better explanation would have been to say that all year long my brain was addled; I cared only about Betty.

Lots of people fall in love in a sensational way. What feels special for Betty and me is that this same love has intensified. It must have been early in our marriage that I woke up one morning and looked at my sleeping partner. In conjunction with my emotions and the rational me, I made a decision: I will love this wonderful and imperfect human being deliberately, conclusively, and permanently. My urge to be with her, my connectedness to her person, and my hope for an uncheckered permanence has never left me.

Betty and I have plenty of things we feel differently about. Even after sixty years, Betty may say something, and I think: she can't believe that! But she does, and together we have to sort out the challenge this difference creates. This proves possible because both of us clutch to a sense of goodwill. We both hate the energy that is spent in our painful attempts to resolve differences, but it's always worth it. What can be better than to share life with someone whom you have every reason to trust, and a span of years behind you that guarantees the reliability and attractiveness of both partners?

Canadians are well-known for their willingness to compromise at world political levels. Betty and I also maintain the steadiness of a long friendship through give-and-take. This is neither a trick nor an easy answer. It requires persistent effort, common sense and commitment. And the exercise of loving.

Teaching Myself How to Teach

Beginnings are always difficult, and learning how to teach was no exception. At the age of nineteen, I was suddenly in charge of twenty-eight kids, Grades One to Nine, in a one-room country schoolhouse five miles north of Winkler, Manitoba. I had learned from both my father and my brother how to tell a story, I had spent a year in Normal School (now Manitoba Teachers College) learning more about Betty Tiessen than about teaching, and now I was expected to become familiar with all Department of Education curricula, Grades One to Eight, and to teach this all in one crowded room. One year too late, I wondered just what I should actually do. It was going to be quite a ride.

I couldn't have asked for more cooperative and decent youngsters, all of whom were ready to learn. They came from homes where the teacher was always considered right. Parents' high expectations of children's schoolwork was the norm. Discipline problems didn't exist. None of the kids was either gifted or slow. At home, television was a new piece of furniture. Only two students had travelled and that was from a Mexican village to Winkler. Every child spent Sunday morning in Sunday school. Lovely kids, all of them.

I initiated a seating plan, placing students in the same grade next to each other. The Grade One pupils sat in front of the room and in front of the three Grade Eight girls who were going to help me teach the little ones how to read. Since the two Grade Nine pupils were taking correspondence, I assigned them to the back of the room. The remaining students sat crammed in the space left. My sweet little grade one boy, Isaac from Mexico, watched with his mouth open. "Full," he said.

I started with a few tried-and-true experiments. After my "Everybody's welcome" spiel I tried a few jokes. No one laughed. I got the students started by assigning various readings to the older ones while I worked directly with the youngest.

It proved impossible to give everyone the attention they needed, but by using the eager Grade Eight girls, there were days when we succeeded. Older students soon became familiar with the long-term goals of their curriculum and, if capable, soon worked on their own.

The Grade Eight pupils seemed to agree with me that, except for new material, their own learning could be enhanced by helping me teach the youngest children in this setting, which offered far too many grades and too little space.

I knew enough to give a great deal of attention to the beginners. Early grounding was by far the most important thing that happened in this wee space with expectations so huge that no single teacher could possibly reach them. But everybody tried.

Evenings

Evenings belonged to Betty. She faced many of the same challenges I did, just seventeen miles south, but with much greater expertise. For fear of exaggerating my love fervour, it might be better to say I picked her up only some evenings during the week, and each weekend. She had most considerate landlords, and I was living at home where my parents never expressed concern about how late I routinely stayed out. I told Jack on one of our rare get-togethers how civil and wise it was of Mama and Papa to ignore what time their nineteen-year-old son came home at night.

Jack said, "Nonsense. Their insight's no better than it ever was. You're the youngest of thirteen and they're just tired." Whatever the cause of their relaxed attitude, I was relieved because there was nothing that could have made me yield even a minute of time spent with Betty.

Engagement

While we were still in our teens, it became clear to us that we would marry. To formalize and speed up this event, my teacher friend Henry Loewen and I drove to Winnipeg and picked up engagement rings we had ordered wholesale through Papa's jeweller friend. The month's salary we each paid to the Winnipeg wholesaler seemed almost too little for such a big event, and we happily forked it over.

On an autumn evening, with the moon shining through the car windows, I fished the expensive-looking box from my pocket, and opened it. Betty and I had promised ourselves to each other long ago, but asking the big question with the ring sparkling in its open box, and hearing Betty's affirmative answer, helped me recognize the moment's magnitude. The hair on the back of my neck never stood straighter. This was for keeps.

When we finally headed for Betty's boarding place that night Betty said, "My dad expects to be asked if he agrees that we get married."

I had expected this. "Can you arrange a time for him and me to get together?" I asked. She nodded.

On the designated evening I drove up the long driveway of the farm where Mr. Tiessen, all alone, was harvesting the final crop of his farming career. His greeting was friendly, and I had learned from Betty how to answer good evening in Low German, a language I had been exposed to but didn't speak well. I had memorized the next words, "Betty and I would like to get married, and thought it proper to get your consent."

He said, "OK. After all, you're a teacher," as though satisfied that I would be able to take good care of his daughter. I managed my part of our chat not too badly, but for the balance of the evening I chose to say no more than I had to, although I did mention that Betty would like to organize an engagement party at their house before Christmas. He nodded.

The engagement party was a celebratory and anticipatory event. We invited some of our best friends who lived not too far away from Gretna, as well as a few more who lived further away. Everyone had a happy evening filled with plenty of jokes about newlyweds. When the last guests had left, and I was putting on my jacket, Betty's dad quietly said to me, "I didn't mean *this* Christmas." He neither smiled nor frowned, and it remained a mystery whether he was making a joke or was displeased at what he perceived to be a rush to get married. I never troubled to find out what he meant. There was no way we would have waited for anybody.

Our Wedding

We were married in Betty's home church set in a pretty Mennonite village west of Gretna. The ceremony included Preacher Friesen's German sermon and the Tiessens' former neighbour and friend Reverend J. K. Klassen married us. We will never forget the choir, an extraordinary amalgamation of our sisters, brothers, and their spouses. Sixty years later we easily recall the tune and the words, and are touched when we remember the excellent rendition.

We spoke our wedding vows, and a typically scrumptious Mennonite *Faspa* was offered to the two hundred guests. The whole event was so masterfully planned that I still joke with Betty, "Had we not shown up, they would have had it anyway!"

Post-Wedding Year

The reality of living together struck like a kind judge's gavel specifying the ruling: guilty on three counts – guilty of having made the biggest of all of life's decisions, guilty of having made the right decision, and guilty of being so lucky! We were so happy together in those few years living in Morden that we couldn't wait to wake up in the early morning when reality's whisper, "It's really true!" sharpened senses we didn't know existed.

Rose beds without thorns don't exist, and we learned early that loving and selfishness are the inevitable coupling that goes with living together, especially if the intention is to be partners of equal worth and wisdom.

Our first year threw numerous curves at us, most of which we knocked deep into the outfield. Ken's birth, our first baby, was a home run, and much more happened to make us happy. My parents loved Betty on the spot. My uncles and aunts wondered out loud how I had made such a "catch." We established new friends at my church. I enjoyed my initiation into high school teaching in Morden Collegiate Institute where we met Dianne and Keith Cooper. They became intimate, life-long friends, and graciously taught us how to begin dealing with our naivety. It seemed nothing could go wrong.

Much later in our marriage we would discover that grief, as deep as joy, could penetrate a family, and that death's intrusion could grasp the initial offspring of life and loving.

Building Our Morden House

While teaching Grade Five in Winkler shortly before Kenny was born, I gave my students a Differential Aptitude Test. I administered it to myself after school. The test confirmed my suspicion that I was all thumbs when it came to any kind of hammer and nails project. Of all the people who had taken the same test, 97% had scored *better* than I had. Failing wasn't something I was used to; I had forgotten how bad it felt.

Embarrassed, I showed it that evening to Betty. She shrugged at my score and laughed a little. "Be glad you're not used to it," she said.

In defiance of my low, low score, I suggested to Betty that we should build a house. Our own house. We were twenty-two years old, and it sounded crazy, even to us, but that night we decided to do it.

It was easy for us to get a loan from the Winkler Credit Union. "After all, you're teachers, aren't you?" said the Winkler Credit Union manager, smiling.

We weren't sure what contractors did. "Organize the building of the building," Betty said, and we decided to do that ourselves. We'd buy a lot from Papa (a double lot, Betty said), then work day and night over the summer months. Finally, and maybe most important, we'd solicit lots of help from relatives and friends – especially from my teaching buddy Henry Loewen, whom we would hire. "Not much time," said Betty. "We better get with it."

"At this point it's still just an idea," I said.

"A whole lot of ideas," Betty added, and I grinned wryly in agreement.

The next Sunday afternoon Papa and I worked out a deal for buying two lots. He wanted to give the land to us, but I wanted to make sure my siblings didn't feel we were being favoured, so we arrived at a price we both liked. Betty, her initiative blossoming, drove to Dack's Pharmacy that same day and brought home half a dozen huge pieces of manilla tag. "Keep the receipt, please," I said, not at all sure we needed to. She nodded and sharpened a pencil, and I found a wooden yardstick. We flattened the heavy-duty paper onto the floor and drew up a house plan over the area where I once built my fort. Energy and enthusiasm had bubbled quickly, and that's all it took to initiate paper plans for a new house for our family.

Our financial essentials fell into place, and in the late spring of 1961, Henry Loewen and I set the pegs which ensured our house would be properly aligned with the street. The critical mind was clearly Henry's, who had terrific mechanical aptitude. We hired professionals when we had to, asked our volunteers for time commitments, and the house grew like Kenny-to-be, very quickly. Betty and I lived at Mama and Papa's place for the summer where the two women canned raspberries and did all the summery things that our female ancestors did for centuries, often without notice or thanks.

We made great progress. When I visited the house fifty-seven years later, it seemed like yesterday that my friends and relatives and I poured the concrete footing, and the house became a wooden duplicate of the manilla tag drawings Betty and I sketched a few months earlier.

Kenny's Birth

On August 17, 1961, Betty woke me at 2:00 a.m. "I'm having pains," she said. I threw on my clothes while she dressed, seemingly at ease. I stood by the door waiting and jingling my car keys.

"Who's the one having the baby?" Betty asked and smiled at my excitement.

I picked up the suitcase which she had prepared months ago for this night and headed for the door. "Let's go," I said.

"Help me down the stairs, please," she said, and I slowed down. A little.

Once outside, I put the suitcase on the driveway beside the car and helped her in. I ran to my side and jumped behind the wheel and pulled the door shut.

"The suitcase," Betty said, and I got out, retrieved it, and threw it into the back seat.

"You've forgotten," said Betty as I spun the wheels. "It usually takes a while for a baby to be born, and it's only seven miles to the hospital." Then she moaned. "Oh! That hurts." She breathed deeply and, after a few minutes she leaned back and relaxed. I didn't.

I had always wanted an excuse to cruise through a stop sign. When we reached Highway 3, I looked left and turned onto the pavement without stopping. I had also always wanted a reason to drive really fast on a main road, but I restrained myself.

The nurse tucked Betty into a white bed in the maternity ward and left for a minute. I finally relaxed a little and kissed Betty goodbye much longer than some folks would have thought necessary.

"They'll call you when the baby's born," she said.

"Good luck," I said, and felt silly because I sounded as though she were off to play a baseball game. I kissed her one last time.

At last I felt I could relax, and I admired the freshly swathed fields of grain drying on the stubble on either side of the highway. From a seed to maturity in a few months, I thought, and the reality of my life suddenly struck me. A baby was about to arrive. Goose bumps stood on my arms. Alone in the car, I smiled and stepped on the accelerator – just a little bit.

The hospital phoned at nine-thirty when I was still asleep. "Mr. Neufeld, you are the father of a healthy baby boy!" the nurse exclaimed.

"Really?" I said as if I were completely surprised. I almost said, "What's his name?" but I collected myself and said, "How's his mother?"

"She's groggy from the anaesthetic, but she'll be fine."

"When can I come see her? Now?"

"This afternoon would be better. She'll be more awake then."

"I'll do that," I said, and hung up the phone. My goose bumps came back. *"Oh, thank you, God,"* I prayed out loud. *"I can't believe it's actually real! Thank you!"*

Betty thinks it's a good thing we can't discern the future. Kenny's arrival was filled with splendid times of new joy, but we knew nothing of the pain we would share with him. Blind to the future, we were spared the anticipatory grieving and the deepest mourning. Our inability to anticipate catastrophic events spared us much pain.

Kenny brought a particular warmth into our home, and an atmosphere of completion. It was marvellous to watch the daily development of a totally new human being, the initiation of a fresh personality.

The baby began his early years in the house that Betty and Hank (and friends) built. In early September 1961, we three moved in, even though the only space completely ready was Kenny's toddler-sized bedroom. During the day, our two-week-old baby spent the autumn days propped up by pillows on the living room couch while his mother painted the walls around him, and our new sound system gave him his first taste of good quality music.

AGE TWENTY-THREE TO TWENTY-NINE

Smoke Signals

After our marriage in 1960, Betty and I moved to Morden where we attended the church I grew up in. Betty was quickly accepted by my parents, and pleasantly received by my relatives and friends. We had both been active in our respective churches and continued volunteering. Betty, an accomplished musician, practised her gift; I taught Sunday school.

Although painfully naive, I was invited to join the Church Council. Thinking that I might represent a perspective that would help balance the views of the older members, I agreed.

The Church Council met on a cool evening in the autumn of 1964. As I parked our blue VW on the church yard, a robin sang in the trees. The bird sounded sad, and I wondered if this was a goodbye signal. I walked into church.

The church sanctuary was reserved mostly for Sunday morning worship, so we met in the basement. Someone had opened a window to help freshen the air, and we kept our jackets buttoned. I knew each of the eight men who were sitting in a circle, but my youthfulness made me feel vulnerable. I felt uncomfortable, and even a little scared.

Preacher Friesen welcomed us and spoke with a quiet authority. He introduced me to the committee, the men raised a hand in greeting, and our leader prayed, asking for guidance.

We dealt quickly with a few practical items. A donation designated for gravelling the parking had been sent, and a member volunteered to write a note of thanks. Someone spoke on behalf of a woman in our congregation who asked to buy a burial site beside her dead husband, and a board member pointed out there was no cost because the graveyard belonged to the congregation. Preacher Friesen produced a calendar and we confirmed *Vierteljahresfest*, a Sunday set aside for thanks to God with all-day services.

"Well," he said, "That part was easy. Now to deal with a more difficult matter. Sad and serious." His lower lip trembled. "Mr. Schmidt, whom we all know, continues to smoke tobacco." Someone coughed. "Congregation members have smelled cigarette smoke on his clothing. Also, someone came unexpectedly upon him recently when he had a cigarette in his mouth." The room was totally still. "He often partakes of a sinful activity. Tonight we must decide what to do."

Through the open window a woodpecker pecked on the wooden siding. The drumming interrupted our concentration, and a few men frowned. Preacher Friesen said, "Now even the birds want in." He turned to me. "Brother Henry, would you chase it away, please." I jumped up, ran outside and threw a stone, and it flew off.

I ran back in time to hear a man ask, "What must we do?"

Somebody else said, "The question is *when* are we going to do it. The Bible tells us if a brother is found to be in habitual sin, two others must visit him and admonish him. If the sinning man refuses to cease, he must be excommunicated."

Excommunicated? I was thunderstruck. The proposed punishment – hell – scarcely fit the misdeed. I had studied *Crime and Punishment,* and this wasn't right. I wondered if I should say something. Shyness was not my dominant trait, but I hesitated. I felt uncertain.

"Correct," agreed a board member, "If that's what the Bible says, then that is what we must do."

I said loudly, "For sucking on burning tobacco?"

"Now, now, Brother Henry," said another member with a white mustache, "there is no need to get excited. You must still learn that being faithful to the Word is always the answer. If the Word is clear, then we must do it."

"But," I said, "if he's excommunicated, doesn't that mean he won't go to heaven?"

"Yes. We are on solid ground," said someone else. "Our body is the temple of the Holy Spirit and it must be treated with respect and dignity. A Christian who smokes is defiling his temple."

All of the men nodded, and I spoke more quietly. "For smoking the leaves of a tobacco plant you're going to excommunicate a man and send him to hell?" No one answered, and the silence became uncomfortable.

Preacher Friesen looked at me for a long minute. Finally, he said, "This council has a tradition. If any board member has a particular concern about a decision we are about to make, we honour his convictions and leave the matter to our next meeting. We needn't decide today."

He turned to the others. "We have asked young Brother Henry to serve on this council and we recognize his legitimacy. We won't decide today. Meanwhile we must speak extreme caution to Brother Schmidt, warning him that he must cease the smoking habit, or we will ask the congregation to excommunicate him. Now, who will caution him?"

Two men raised their hands, Preacher Friesen spoke their names and closed the meeting with a prayer. He asked God to help Brother Schmidt cease his sinful habit and his voice broke. He gathered himself and continued, "Lest his sinful habit destroy his very soul."

The group dissolved and, astonished and strangely sad, I wanted to cry. "Come, Brother Henry," Preacher Friesen said, getting to his feet. "You have seen that some choices we make are extremely difficult and sometimes have harsh consequences. But we have Scripture on our side, and so this decision is right." I stood up and he put his arm around my shoulders, and we walked out of the basement together.

Pete, Marion, Disaster

When he was in his twenties, my oldest brother Pete married gentle Marian Hart from Boissevain. Although he and Marian had four lovely children, and although he became a successful lumber yard manager, Pete's life was dominated by alcohol addiction. He managed to function as an active alcoholic for several decades. The liquid curse obsessed him.

In the mid '60s he finally lost his job. Jack and I borrowed brother-in-law Albert's farm truck and moved the family to our parents' cold and empty house in Morden. That winter, Pete and his family became familiar with privation and, by Canadian standards, they approached destitution.

Just before Easter they scraped together, from piggy banks and pockets, enough loose change to take a bus to Boissevain, Marian's home. There, while in her mother's kitchen stirring gravy, standing among her four children, Marian experienced a blood clot. Her aneurism was instant and fatal.

After Marian's funeral, crisis decisions had to be made quickly. Marian's parents took home the two girls. Pete took David and Stanley back to Morden.

His craving for alcohol proved too strong for Pete's disposition, and this took its toll on the two boys. No one knew what they actually ate. They were often away from school. They had cold sores on their faces. Unless Betty and I dropped in, they spent their evenings alone, and went to bed alone. Pete was seldom home.

Betty and I thought long and carefully about taking David into our family. We spoke to my sister Marion and her husband Al and decided to talk to Pete about it.

I approached him. "I don't want to offend you, Pete," I said, "but you must know your boys aren't doing very well."

"So," he said, "what am I supposed to do about it?" Although only thirty-nine years old, his lined face and pale-blue eyes looked tired and stressed.

"We have a proposition." I spoke with trepidation because I was talking to my oldest brother about taking his kids away from him.

"Meaning?" he asked.

I spoke quickly. "Betty and I would happily accept David into our home. I've talked to Marion and Al and they agree to take Stanley." I added awkwardly, "If you agree."

Pete stared into the distance for what seemed a full minute. Then he looked at me. "OK," he said, and walked away. The next day we picked up David and took him and his personal belongings to his new home – ours.

I began reading books about the power of addiction. I knew nothing about alcoholism except that it had cost Pete his job, his four children, and, probably, his wife. He had loved Marian deeply, he adored his children, and his management job was his family's only livelihood. Why would anyone choose to give up all that in exchange for maintaining daily, heavy alcohol consumption? Beats me, I thought.

I had heard somewhere that addiction involved an element of helplessness. Even in 1911 some researchers concluded that alcoholism was a disease which actually caused a loss of personal choice. Was it possible for Pete to choose differently? Should alcoholism be viewed more like an illness? If so, a community's pejorative way of speaking about the "town drunk," or as an irresponsible lout, might be quite unfair. These thoughts put me on the road to better understand Pete, although they did little to prepare me for a future heavy with loss directly related to addiction.

David, Son and Brother

Pete's sad and alienated life was our first introduction to the power of addiction. Addiction's capacity to cause a rational person to give up everything he loves for a life governed by booze bewildered us. We hadn't the slightest notion that eventually we would come to know the nature of alcohol all too well.

Kenny's single bed was shoved against the wall and a bed for David slid against it. A fourth place was added to our dining room table, and overnight we had a second boy and Kenny had a brother. David's abrupt losses of mother, father, and three siblings must have penetrated each pathway of his new life like sharp knives. But we were excited to have him, and he soon called us Mom and Dad and we introduced him to our friends as our son.

Work and studies took our new family from Morden to Waterloo, Ontario, to Minnedosa and then to Thompson. Everything must have felt novel for David: toys, clothes, school, church, friends, even his mom and dad and brother were brand new. But he was a good fit.

By a dreadful coincidence, David's family losses were almost identical to Grandpa Neufeld's seventy years ago. David had lost his mother and all his siblings inside of a week; his father disappeared from his life a week later.

At nine, David was shy and self-effacing: he tried always to please. Betty and I were twenty-six, and totally naive in matters of a child's grief, but we constantly encouraged David. "You're not a visitor," we coaxed. "This is your home. You're one of us." We hoped that our multiple hugs could lead to trust, and that our gentle words would calm his anxieties. No matter how hard we worked to make him feel comfortable and accepted, however, he was a nervous child, overly willing to please. David's sudden loss of his family left nasty scars in his heart, and loneliness became his partner.

Mennonite Brethren Bible College

For a long time, I believed attending Mennonite Brethren Bible College in Winnipeg would be the year I would seal my commitment toward a life of "serving the Lord." It would be a time of consolidation, of recognizing the call of God. This year of study would help me choose more precisely the theological work toward which I would direct my life.

This would not be unusual. Many graduates of MBBC held positions as missionaries, ministers, Bible School teachers, and many other career choices directly related to the church. This, however, didn't happen to me.

Early in my first full year at a post-secondary institution, I asked the librarian at the MBBC for a work written by Paul Tillich, probably the most well-known Protestant theologian of the century. He said, "We don't carry books by Paul Tillich." Startled, I asked why, and was informed that Tillich was too liberal a theologian to be carried by MBBC. I was in my early twenties but relatively well-read – enough to know that for my church college not to carry Paul Tillich was a punch in the face of a most-respected contemporary Christian theologian. I was amazed.

The fact that the library at MBBC didn't carry Paul Tillich reminded me of how the Roman Catholics had created an Index which identified the books Catholics were permitted to read, and the ones they weren't. I had learned early on to admire and highly respect my college professors, but this event turned out to be a watershed experience. Daring to come to my own position, I concluded that at the highest polity level, our church's college differed so greatly from my own thinking, that I wondered what other things of negative theological import I would discover at MBBC.

I spent the morning of our Day of Fasting contemplatively. Not eating for a day created a surprising amount of time because it eliminated cleaning up, preparing food and eating it. I had time to contemplate, read and pray. By mid-afternoon I quite suddenly came to a clear understanding about an issue that I had struggled with for years: I realized that I no longer believed the Bible was the literal, unerring word of God.

This had huge implications for my spiritual life, so I looked up Dr. Adrian, my history professor. He was an outstanding teacher whose logic and consistency defined his teaching. He demonstrated clear perspectives, and willingly admitted the particular biases he adhered to.

Today, when I spelled out my serious questions about the Bible being the unerring, literal Word of God, he looked startled.

"But," he said, "the Bible itself testifies to that."

"I know that," I said. "I know the Bible claims its own authenticity."

"So," said Dr. Adrian, "isn't that enough for you?"

"No," I said. "Not at all."

"Brother," he said, "in the second book of Timothy we read 'All Scripture is given by inspiration.' Isn't that enough for you?"

Dr. Adrian was not only an excellent professor, but he was also an honourable man and honest thinker. In History class, when success-fully challenged, he lacked defensiveness and freely acknowledged his errors. So I told him that I knew he would never claim that a given piece of historical information was true because it said it was. So, on what basis, I asked, did he treat the Scriptures differently? He was silent for a long minute. I added, "For example, I'm sure you wouldn't claim that Shakespeare's works are God's unerring words just because Polonius said they were."

"No," he said, "I wouldn't."

We spoke for an hour and, in the end, I concluded that here was a learned man of integrity who, for whatever reason, excluded the

Bible from his list of books whose assumptions his professionalism demanded he examine – just like he would any other text. Surprised at my professor's abrupt reversal in logic, and very disappointed, I felt a pronounced shift in my religious belief system; perhaps it marked the beginning of a new consolidation.

I walked home. Kenny was sleeping. Betty and I finished our schoolwork. Then we talked a long time about our religious beliefs, and just how and what we intended to teach Kenny about God.

From what she said, it was clear that Betty never had the intensity of religious struggle that I did. The leadership in her church placed a less rigid emphasis on recognizing right from wrong. Her Mennonite church took strong positions on critical issues of truth and untruth, but they seemed more reluctant to declare themselves certain in arguable areas of right and wrong. Rather than pontificate, they made distinctions.

I had always believed Betty's church conference to be overly patient when facing decisions which I thought called for promptitude, but now I wasn't so sure. Her Mennonite church accepted the grace of God through Jesus as axiomatic, but they adhered to specific and difficult issues with a quiet humility. Rather than follow my father's tormented cry, "*Ich bin so schlecht*" [I am so bad], they trusted in God's unconditional love for all humankind, no terms attached.

It seemed a peculiar irony, I thought, that the Mennonite Brethren Church, often judgmental of other churches, declared God's love as unconditional. Could they have it both ways? How contradictory to proclaim God's unconditional love for everyone while maintaining an absolute primacy on having a strictly defined conversion experience. Was it possible to honour the Spirit while insisting on contradictory logic?

Jesus admonished his disciples to think simply, as little children do, to maintain a child*like* attitude, not a child*ish* way of thinking. When he was a child, said Paul, he thought like a child, but when he became a man, he thought like an adult. Put away child*ish* things, he said. Far, far better to practise a child*like* humility than to emulate a child*ish* way of thinking.

Minnedosa: Morden Rejection

In 1968 we moved to Minnedosa, Manitoba, a town lying in a beautiful valley. We felt great excitement to find our terrific friends, Dianne and Keith Cooper, waiting for us.

Minnedosa had a wonderful rural air. Saturday night every store was open until ten, and in good weather the streets and sidewalks were crowded with farmers' vehicles; groups of people chatted amiably on every street corner, and in front of every establishment. The grocery stores made a considerable percentage of their week's sales in the last four hours of Saturday as farm folks hauled their supply of brown-bagged groceries to their vehicles. Here and there, dogs sniffed around for eatable items, but even they were tail-wagging friendly.

Among the main streets of various business establishments stood an impressive old building. Although unlit and empty on Saturday night, the busy streets seemed an appropriate place for what was Minnedosa's United Church.

Betty attended here almost as soon we arrived and was particularly attracted to the light and lovely sound of the church's children's choir. She quickly became director Jean Stephenson's piano accompanist. This brought me back to regular church attendance and, after a year, we decided to become members. I wrote my home church, Morden Mennonite Brethren, asking for a church transfer. Our old church's response caused Betty and me utter astonishment.

The Morden Mennonite Brethren Church, which I had been born into, where I experienced a child conversion, where I experienced a happy baptism, where I had felt an intense sense of belonging, the church which I loved, indicated "No" to our request for a transfer. Their letter said the Mennonite Brethren Church granted transfers "only to churches of like faith." We were totally taken aback, and deeply saddened. Ironically, the letter helped to affirm our decision to change churches.

I wrote back asking the Morden Mennonite Brethren Church to strike our names from its membership list. The personal warmth which greeted us in our new church, and the eagerness with which our new denomination welcomed our contributions, meant that we were happy there.

We tried not to let our hurt turn to anger, but it was difficult not to feel unfairly criticized by a church which believed the Bible literally, including Jesus' warning, "Do not judge."

Years later I visited Preacher Friesen (nearly one hundred years old then). Recalling this formal rejection, he wept and said, "We have made many mistakes." Indeed, they had. Leaving the only church I had ever known created a scenario of ongoing chagrin.

Jacquie's Birth

After Kenny's birth in Morden, Betty's doctor said it was unlikely that she would be pregnant again. He said something about a narrow pelvis. In March of 1968 Betty told me the doctor was indisputably wrong. Joy and I jumped like African antelopes. For seven years we had hoped for another youngster, and when we told our two boys, all of us shouted, even Kenny and David who, at seven and eleven, didn't quite get it.

Betty bought the fluffiest curtains Minnedosa had in stock, she wallpapered Jacquie's room, and somewhere she found a bassinette and upgraded it from pretty to "Oh, so cute!"

At Home with Jacquie

Each of us was drawn to the tiniest room in our house where we studied Jacquie's rotund baby face and marvelled at her tininess. A sense of well-being permeated every room, every corner, even the sink where we washed dishes. The boys' delight showed itself in ways we hadn't seen before. Our home was swamped with happiness. Kenny and David satisfied themselves with gentle pokes to the baby's lips, trying to make them curl up in a smile. I hadn't quite anticipated such unlimited enthusiasm. Awe had struck.

Seven-year-old Kenny had one reservation. After trying to get Baby Jacquie to play with him, and she just lay there, he said, "But she can't *do* anything." His minor complaint turned out to be premature because Jacquie turned out to be a do-er with loads of energy and ability.

I had a concern about a new baby in the house. "A man's heart is only the size of his closed fist," I said to Betty privately. "That's not very big. Do you think I have room for loving you and the boys as well as the new baby? My heart might be overcrowded."

"You old romantic," laughed Betty. "Don't worry. Your heart will grow." She smiled at the baby, and threw me a kiss.

Jacquie Grows Up

Jacquie, of course, grew up as the family baby. She had two older brothers who may have thought she would remain "baby," but they were in for a surprise. Jacquie owned a sense of resolution which became a motivating force in her life. Once, when she was ten, she emphatically but politely stood up to her mother, and I told her, "Way to go, Jacquie! If you can stand up to your mother, you'll be able to confront most anybody." Betty smiled, and gave Jacquie a big hug.

Six years later, working as a waitress, an angry fellow employee addressed Jacquie in terms that were demeaning and quite unrepeatable. Jacquie promptly got him and their boss together, and repeated word for word what had been said to her, adding, "Nobody talks like that to me outside this restaurant, and nobody's going to talk to me like that inside this place, either." The supportive boss eyed Jacquie, nodded, and took the employee into the next room – and Jacquie's self-respecting personality was established in the workplace.

I was delighted to hear this, relieved that nobody was going to push our daughter around, or treat her badly without an effective reprisal. It was one less worry for my fatherly mind.

Jacquie attended Westgate Collegiate, a Mennonite high school that gave her a lifetime habit of taking her schooling seriously. She also developed delightful friendships with level-headed and life-loving friends at the school.

After Jacquie earned a Bachelor of Arts degree, the desire for travel carried her to Australia. In nearby New Zealand she met David Johnson, and a few years later a wedding was in the offing. Two grandchildren, Rebekah and Charlie, followed quickly and this remarkable family eventually moved to Winnipeg and bought a house fifteen minutes from our home.

As a schoolgirl, Jacquie hadn't shown remarkable tendencies toward academic achievement. That made her later success all the more noteworthy as she earned a Master of Education degree.

She moved from working as a classroom teacher to becoming a language support teacher, a specialty profession where she assisted classroom teachers who taught special needs children. Having written about the development of her career, it feels strange for me to note that she qualifies for retirement in 2024.

PART II

My Names

Henry, Heina, Hank, Edward, Eddy, Ed

If it's true that one's sense of self is closely related to one's name, I should be a confused man. My parents affixed Henry Edward to my birth certificate, but everybody called me Hank, and Mama gave me the affectionate German nickname Heina.

Martha took me to school the first day of Grade One. She didn't like the sound of Hank or Henry, so she told Miss McFadden my name was Edward. Only a year later my new teacher, Miss Lawsen, thought Edward sounded too grown-up, so she scratched out Edward and printed Eddy. I was called Eddy until Mr. James in junior high thought Ed sounded more like a young man's name. His end-of-year report confused my high school teachers, and most called me Edward. My Grade Twelve certificate went full circle and officially identified me as Henry Edward Neufeld. My siblings and friends continued to call me Hank. I tried to eliminate this confusion at Manitoba Teachers College by registering as my friends knew me, Hank, but the college registrar would accept only my birth certificate as identification, and it said Henry Edward.

It's not true that name confusion affects one's sense of identity. Rather, it confuses teachers. Twenty years after high school, I ran into Miss Lawsen, then a resident in the Morden Old Folks' Home. I was very pleased to see her.

"Hi, Miss Lawsen," I said.

She looked at me carefully. "If it isn't Billy Friesen from Morden," she finally said, "How you've grown!"

Gardewine Trucking

At nineteen, I started teaching. This early start on a pension plan meant I was able to retire at fifty-six.

The first school day in September found me reading the *Winnipeg Free Press* and feeling guilty because a delivery truck passing by reminded me that today was a workday, and here I sat with my feet up, reading a newspaper. This new reality felt strange, but exciting. I wasn't shocked enough not to be able to adjust the pillow behind my back, sip my cup of coffee, and grin at the cognitive dissonance I felt.

I hadn't finished reading a section of the paper before Gardewine Trucking of Winnipeg called to ask me to conduct a job satisfaction survey of their truck drivers. While I didn't need to work for money anymore, I had ample energy to take on an interesting-sounding new job. I began in October 1995.

Rather than the usual series of written questions, a summary of the workers' answers, and my written recommendations, I wanted my satisfaction survey results to reflect a more accurate summary than such a procedure entailed. Instead of following the common paper route, I visited every Gardewine Trucking Station by air or by car (thirty-one such bases stretched from Calgary to Toronto, from Morden to Churchill.) I visited places I would otherwise never have encountered, and interviewed every person who drove a company truck. From the records I kept of interviews with the truckers who worked for Gardewine truckers, I wrote a Summary Satisfaction Survey before the end of the year. The work was exciting, and every day I met interesting people.

Volunteer Activities

Working on Four Boards

New Directions

New Directions works with clients who present the most difficult people problems in Winnipeg. In the year 2000, this government-funded organization had an annual budget of twelve million dollars.

I volunteered seven terms as member, vice chair, chair, and past chair. I had long felt a particular empathy for what was then called Children's Home because my good friend Keith Cooper worked there as chief executive officer, and had kept me connected with the organization's activities. I enjoyed the responsibilities the board work entailed; setting new policy and reviewing old was part of the work I enjoyed most. The board often got involved with current crises and long-term public relations. Some days the work felt like a half-time job – and I loved it.

John Howard Society

Named after its founder, the society's task is to act as an advocacy group for prisoners. I was hugely inspired. As chair of the organization, I learned how prisons operate. (The short answer to that is "poorly".) For a term I was a board member of the Canadian association as well, and what I learned from the organization's top people convinced me how ineffective and even harmful incarceration frequently is.

Stony Mountain Penitentiary Volunteer Visitor

After leaving the John Howard Society board, I volunteered at Stony Mountain Penitentiary as a prison-designated "friend" to a particular prisoner who had no friends or family visiting him during his seventeen-year prison sentence. This marvellous, eye-opening experience lasted over a three-year period. During my biweekly visits, a certain trust and liking developed between us, and I learned much, much more about the day-to-day life of a prisoner than I could have possibly picked up in my board work. My friend, a middle-aged man, will be released soon, and he is as ready to step into our technological society as I am prepared to be a prisoner at Stony Mountain Penitentiary!

Fort Garry United Church

Betty and I joined the Fort Garry United Church, Winnipeg in 1983. Betty became involved in the music department of the church, and I began some committee work. Our stay has been rewarding, especially the regular discussion groups made up of individuals who have become our friends. I also served four years as a member and then as chair of the church council.

Organization for Cooperation in Overseas Development

After retirement, Betty and I volunteered for two winters in Caribbean schools which were in need of counsel and direction. OCOD was a federal government organization that sent volunteer teachers to a variety of places in the Caribbean, St. Kitts-Nevis and Dominica, in our case. We remember the two locations with satisfaction and lasting fondness.

We also worked an additional winter in Jamaica in a privately run school with equal pleasure.

Travelling

We spent our first honeymoon night in a borrowed, leaky tent on the Whiteshell camping grounds. In itself, this may not sound exciting, but it soon stopped raining. It was a challenging time – in part because we owned no indispensables such as sleeping bags, a lamp, a propane stove, and other camping necessities. This is how we began the first of many tenting expeditions, each exciting in its own way, especially this one. In 1972, twelve years later, Betty's Uncle Jasch died and left a little bundle of cash for each of his nieces and nephews. We thought this perfect timing for buying camping gear, so we shopped for a decent tent and all the accoutrements. We tented in most Canadian provinces, in some U.S. western states, in Germany, Switzerland, Austria, and a few other countries.

Travelling changed us – not our essential selves, but it gave us new perspectives we would not otherwise have developed. We first discovered our pathetic naivety in Haiti in 1967, when a hungry toddler in her mother's arms reached out a hand to me and said, "Nickel?" Haiti was then, and still is, the poorest country in our hemisphere, and the one-year-old obviously hadn't eaten for some time, so I gave the mother some change. In no time, we were sur-rounded by a crowd of adults pushing and shoving towards us shouting, "Money, money!" We had become instant targets, and the Haitians crowded around us, pulling at our shirt sleeves in a desperate, aggressive way, reaching, imploring. Quite frightened, we slipped into a restaurant before any of the hungry Haitians became even more assertive in their loud demands for what they must have regarded as shareable wealth.

This, our first encounter with a crowd of hungry people, stuck in our minds – and especially in our hearts – more effectively than any television image ever could.

In Mexico we once experienced a less dramatic encounter with the poor. In an inconspicuous little town with no group of hungry adults around us, I gave a ragged-looking youngster a dollar. He ran into a nearby shack and raced out with an empty bottle. He ran to a corner store, came out with a full bottle of milk, and hurried back to the shack. "For the baby," he called to us.

Both these incidents, in effect, cost us nothing, and we claim no credit. Rather, it makes me ashamed of our fine condo, where the menu is usually pretty well anything we want. I think back to my financially limited father and how eagerly he gave ten percent to "missions" even when his family then ate more poorly.

I am thankful for the living standard I can afford, but it will always remain one of my life's unresolved conundrums when I consider the huge inconsistency between how most of us Christians talk on Sunday and how we act the rest of the week. From a world view, the contradiction is so hypocritical that – were it not so horrible – the irony is laughable. I imagine a personal God "out there" beyond our space crafts, casting Godly eyes at our globe, and seeing how most of us grow richer while hordes of people suffer and die because the simplest nutrition is not available. What a discredit to us, the so-called emulators of a giving Jesus.

I grew up in a twin-like "Christian" society. One was the society at large; it considered itself "Christian" as compared to, say, "Muslim." The other twin, the Morden Mennonite Brethren Church, for example, preached generosity wherever applicable. My family, while poorer than most, gave proportionately more than many other

Christians. (We had other sins.) The very overweight preachers who wrote their sermons condemning tobacco while overdosing on food had much to answer for.

It's true, just a few of us cannot solve the world's hunger calamity, but nobody's keeping score, and the specific people that are fed by our giving, keeps *them* alive. Jesus didn't advocate ten percent, but rather, everything. The One we claim to emulate, is once more made into a laughingstock. Is it possible that Christians concentrate on ten percent in order to put a Biblical gloss on their giving?

The Billy Connection

My longest personal attachment outside of my family is my friend Bill. This connection has easily survived our living in different parts of the country, and beyond. The first day in Grade One we walked to school and, less regularly, walked together through the next seventy-five years. As adults we live half a continent from each other, but telephone calls, letters by post, notes by e-mail, and regular visits have kept us strongly bonded. One spring, I emailed Bill to say we would have to skip getting together because Betty and I would be in Germany. He wrote back, "Where in Germany?" I answered him, and he came to spend time with us in Munich. That is the nature of our affiliation.

Bill and I grew up a block away from each other and somewhat further apart in our parents' choice of church: I attended the Mennonite Brethren Church and he, albeit having a Mennonite name and background, attended the Pentecostal Church. This distinction mattered nothing at all to us kids, even though the adult linkage between the churches was nil. Papa occasionally visited with Bill's dad, but I know of no other personal fusion between the two churches.

After high school, Bill and I drove off to separate colleges. This interrupted our close connectedness until we were established in our respective professions.

Bill and I took different paths in the area of religion. Over the years I had voiced serious questions about Mennonite dogma, but he left his church permanently. After Betty and I joined the United Church of Canada, I once told him, "You know, you threw out the baby with the bath, while I threw out the bath and kept the baby." He agreed, and we continued to find more things in common than otherwise. I admire Bill's capacity to think rationally. He tries never to come to grips with matters on the basis of emotion, but insists that reason is the only way to truth. In debate, he accepts nothing short of logic.

"But how do you *know* that?" is one of his frequent questions. He hates hypocrisy, both inside and outside religious formations, and despite his rigid stance, I've come to share his views on many things.

It's amazing to me that many differences have never caused our emotional closeness to die off. His is not only my longest friendship, but also the tops in humour and intensity of caring. We laugh lots and loudly and, when Ken died, we wept. I experienced one particular computer exchange after Ken's funeral like a living sympathy card. Computers can do most anything, and this one made me cry.

Bill's influence on me has been constant. The trust we have built allows us to be open with each other. Neither of us is afraid to tell the other what he believes, particularly about life's big questions. Such frankness allows us to be real with each other even when we disagree. This is a gift not easily maintained in a world in which there are many pressures to conform. It allows me now to say with complete comfort, "I love the guy."

Woman Alive

When I think of Betty and me, I think of *before* and *after*. It's as though I've had two lives, one prior to meeting her and one after. She hasn't only been the centre of my life, but rather we are extensions of each other. My basic value system developed before I met her. My family and church greatly affected my adult ethic, but being with Betty for over sixty years profoundly impacted the spirit that moves me.

Betty and the piano were friends long before she met me. Her singing family taught her that life's barren qualities are wonderfully lifted by music. I fell in love with Betty listening to her play the piano in teachers' college one evening when she thought she was alone. The sound produced by her outstanding eye-finger coordination, so poignant as to make me cry, proved to be a talent that touched people wherever she and a piano got together.

Betty executes the demands of her nature which insists on equality. Sometimes it takes the form of feminism, but it is not limited to women's issues. Fairness and justice always dominate the invisible banner she carries.

A reader of a thousand books, Betty delves into serious literature as well as lighter material. As a girl, Betty read the few good books she had at her disposal over and over. As she matured, intellectual treatise and travel books also appealed to her. During retirement, besides reading literally hundreds of books, word puzzles proved to be her forte. I tried a few times to compete, but my efforts proved too draining.

At work, she struck a fine balance between the overly strict teacher and the pedagogue too hasty to switch fads. Betty welcomed new methodologies, but was not quick to invest herself into the unproven. At parties, she was a gas. Betty was also what others called "a tough cookie." She ended her teaching career by resigning mid-year rather than conceding to the school superintendent's refusal to yield five days of unpaid leave to be in England with Jacquie when our first grandchild was born.

Betty's private person appeals most to those who know her best. She is a lover of good jokes and much laughter. Conversely, Betty's colleagues remember her when professional courage needs exemplification.

Comparing the enthusiastic lovely young woman at Manitoba Teachers' College to the spunky older woman she has become, one is struck by both the similarities and differences. Her earlier aliveness turned into a softer enthusiasm. A young person's courage to face a barrage of challenges has settled into a quiet, astute confidence which emerged from multiple years of professional experiences.

Twin family losses had an immense effect on her person when we lost our son Ken and grandson Evan to deadly tragedies a few years ago. Sometimes it seems part of Betty travelled away with them and what is left of her is wiser, deeper, and more sadly beautiful.

Ernest Hemingway said all love stories must end unhappily. He meant that people's death terminates their human feeling. I shiver because I cannot imagine being without Betty. Her absence would take a critical part of me along with her.

I recognize that no relationships are "made in heaven," but for us it often feels that way. Since our wedding sixty years ago, we have so frequently and intensely cried together and loudly laughed together that, even now, a third party, watching from a hidden place, would say that a neutrality of feeling between us is a rarity.

When our son Ken died, and his son, twenty-three-year-old Evan followed suit, we anticipated that the stress and strain would test our marriage to its limit. It did, and yet the disasters drew us closer together, and our commitment to each other swelled. We were reborn into a deeper relationship which freed us to be more fully our individual selves, while adding intimacy and self-revelation to each other.

Betty has been, by far, the most important and influential person in my life. Her strength of character was essential to my emotional survival during turbulent times in my career. Her ability to forgive forged closer ties between us. Her love of life encouraged me to move away from that part of my background that, on reflection, was overly coercive and inhibiting. Like a bird calling from the sky, she lifted me.

Twin Disasters

Kenny, as a Boy

The anxiety Ken showed when he started school in Minnedosa in 1995 concerned us. He could easily hold his own with his young friends – and in adult conversation – but, as he grew older, he told us that the close proximity of others caused a marked increase in his heart rate, accelerated breathing, perspiration, and overall discomfort. This happened to him with each day's personal encounters. We didn't understand that we were witnessing symptoms of social anxiety.

When Kenny was born, my parents lived directly across from our new house in Morden. Papa had retired recently, and he spent hours on the porch rocking Kenny just as he had rocked his dying four-year-old son three decades earlier, in Winkler. Now was a happier time. Papa was more relaxed, he was retired, and the obligation of feeding a large family was no longer the driving force in his life. Kenny cooed and smiled in Papa's arms; their relationship was trustingly sweet.

Kenny was a sensitive little boy who carried an awareness of other people's pain, and went out of his way to alleviate it. As a preschooler, he hovered around me asking what he could do to make my nasty headache better. Kenny's personal sensitivity showed itself in cheerful ways, too. When Betty was eight months pregnant, and walking down our stairway carrying a vase full of roses, with a healthy glow on her cheeks, he said, "Mom, you look just like what you're carrying!"

This touching sensitivity to those around him sometimes showed itself in more crude ways. We once took seven-year-old Kenny to a concert where the music was quite beyond his years. His boredom was broken when I took him with me into the men's washroom during the intermission, where he stared, unbelieving, as I used the urinal. When we came out, he shouted at Betty so she could hear him above the noise of people chattering. "Mommy," he yelled, "Daddy peed against the wall!"

During his preschool age, Kenny loved playing in the wooded area which I had called The Island less than twenty years ago. I made him a makeshift bow and arrow, and he shot at a sparrow. He was only five, and had no hope, or wish, to hit it – but he did. Kenny carried the dead bird into the house and, with a mixture of pride in his marksmanship and grief at having killed a living creature, he cried, "I hit it! I didn't mean to! I didn't mean to – I was just lucky!"

My stomach squirmed as I compared my wonderfully unique experience on The Island with his. As a little boy, playing among the trees and a great variety of birds, 1 was first introduced to the idea of the Sacred. Now, Kenny was crying about a small bird he accidentally killed, surrounded by the very same trees, and on the same spot where I had experienced a profoundly comforting Presence.

"Come here, Kenny," I said, and he came and wrapped his arms around my neck.

"Why are you crying?" he asked me as I hugged him, and licked at the tears flowing past the corners of my mouth.

In Thompson, Manitoba, 1971–1975, playing in a junior baseball league, Ken shone as a pitcher. Whenever I watched him, I remembered how, from age nine to twelve, he and I had played catch with gloves and a hardball. Those were good times for both of us, and now they were paying off.

In his Winnipeg high school, a few years later, Ken excelled at basketball, and missed the provincial playoffs in badminton only because of a strained back. He never bragged about his accomplishments, but he loved sports of any kind, and athletics played a positive role in his development toward adulthood.

Once, at home, I insisted he mow our lawn, and fourteen-year-old Kenny explained his reluctance. "Dad," he said, "I don't have the same investment in the lawn as you do." We quickly resolved that particular difference in aesthetics, he obediently started the lawnmower, and I watched as he improved his appreciation of greenery. He grinned until he was finished.

Kenny was great fun. His sense of humour was keen and, even when he was very young, he loved laughing and telling jokes. In high school, this lightness of living also showed when he did little homework and relied on quick, off-the-cuff answers to get a decent pass. Even in church he knew what to say: one Sunday when he was six and sitting in the pews with us, he kept closing his eyes. I leaned over and suggested he listen to what was being said, but he smiled and waved me off. At home we asked him what he had been doing during the service, wide awake but with his eyes closed. "Watching cartoons," he explained.

Ken, as a Man

Ken told me he had his first alcoholic drink at a Grade Ten high school party. He recollected how his anxiety lifted, his shyness disappeared, and he liked the feeling. A few weeks later, I noticed an unexpected lowering of the level of an opened wine bottle we kept in the fridge. I had also heard glasses tinkling behind his bedroom door, and when I confronted him, he admitted to occasional use. He was fifteen years old, and I directed him to absolutely abstain. He answered that one of his high school buddies drank beer every day. "But not you," I said, my voice emphatic. "That's not negotiable!"

For the next few years, Ken either minimized his drinking or effectively hid it from us. Alcohol consumption at his age worried us profoundly and we hoped, almost desperately, that his lapses in judgment would improve. That wish was eventually shattered like shards of glass from a broken bottle.

After his high school graduation, Ken felt unsure what he wanted to do next, but thought an undergraduate degree in arts would open the door to further study. He adjusted well to university and received a Bachelor of Arts degree.

At David's wedding in 1980, Ken met Elaine, sister to David's new wife. A year later Ken moved in with Elaine and they lived together for nine years before marrying. Their wedding was, Ken told me, the happiest day of his life. This happiness was to be greatly compounded with the birth of their son Evan some years later.

As a youth, Ken used to subscribe to *Psychology Today*, a magazine that played a significant role in his registering in the Selkirk Mental Health Hospital to study a two-year program in psychiatric nursing. He became a successful student, admired for his joy of life and for his maturing mind. At his graduation he won the reward for most popular student, a far cry from the earlier anxiety that had been his companion when he was a boy. No parents were prouder of their adult child than we were of Ken. His psychiatric training led to a career that closely suited his interests and abilities.

Long ago, when I was a high school counsellor in Morden, a teenager once said to me, "What do you mean, 'drugs are bad'? They're good! They take away my miserable thoughts. Problems disappear. Drugs make me happy! Drugs are good."

This comment had a dangerous, superficial truth: Ken himself told us what fine times he had during his early drinking days. His shoulders lightened, he said, and the worries of everyday living evaporated. Alcohol erased his painful anxieties. Drinking was fun! We, of course, pointed out the potential misery and possible lethality of long-term, excessive use.

Ken began drinking more. This corresponded with his securing a job with the Crisis Rehabilitation Unit, an in-patient organization run by the Salvation Army in Winnipeg. The CRU staff dealt with some of the most troubled people in Winnipeg, mostly hardcore addicts with mental health issues. Ken's responsibilities were precisely what he had been trained for, although the irony was not lost on us that Ken shared his clients' addiction problems.

In 1995 when I retired, we became so concerned about Ken's regular drinking that Betty and I sought out intensive and detailed information on the subtleties of addiction. One evening a week, for three months, the two of us attended classes with individuals who shared similar problems in their families, whether alcohol was the addicting drug, or other "hard drugs." Experts in addiction taught us how to support Ken while not unwittingly enabling him in his drinking. We learned that, once addicted, an alcoholic person cannot normally stop drinking without help, any more than he can defeat cancer on his own. The difference is treatment type, addiction being responsive to non-medication individual, or group, treatment. We quickly realized that addiction is a disease, not a matter of personal resolve.

We kept in close touch with Ken, Evan and Elaine, who lived fifteen minutes from our house, but we avoided seeing or speaking to Ken when he wasn't sober. We met him for lunch, visited him, and encouraged him to come visit. On occasion, he spoke openly and frankly of what had become a deadly addiction.

The distinction between supporting Ken and taking a tough stand against his addiction was a subtle one. On the basis of what we had learned, and in a lasting attempt to show consistent compassion, we deliberately adopted a non-judgmental attitude toward the son we loved. While never acting in ways that made his drinking easier (like giving him money), Betty and I worked hard at retaining an open, loving attitude toward him. We hated his alcohol addiction, but we did not view Ken himself as bad. Our commitment to him and his family remained unconditional. We remained non-judgmental of his person, but not of the addiction, and, in a moment of candour and sobriety, he told us that our unambiguous attitude helped him to be open with us when discussing his alcoholism, but the level of anxiety his addiction caused everyone was extreme.

Despite our doing everything possible, Ken's heavy drinking continued. He kept his psychiatric nursing job by being careful never to go to work inebriated. He developed, and then held, his excellent work reputation. Colleagues looked to him for direction in emergencies, and novice nurses depended on him for learning to understand the practical function of a Crisis Rehabilitation Unit. Hospital psychiatrists trusted Ken's judgments and, as he developed into a veteran and respected psychiatric nurse, they depended on him to cover for them when necessary. He enjoyed his professional reputation and somehow maintained it.

We made a decision to avoid being secretive about Ken's addiction to alcohol, and to share Ken's status with our friends. Our shame subsequently faded, and our friends' support in emulating our attitude of non-judgment toward Ken became open and direct. Mutual sharing was a godsend.

Leadership vacancies at work were frequently advertised, and Ken's colleagues encouraged him to apply but, knowing his personal limitations, he stayed where his addiction was least noticeable, and where expectations fit his aptitudes. He maintained his professional reputation, even while admitting to us that he was a functioning alcoholic.

At Ken and Elaine's home addiction took a heavy toll. The stresses put the marriage at risk, and divorce resulted. Soon young Evan spent one week with his mother and the next with his father. All three found the separation which their divorce made necessary increasingly difficult. Evan suffered acutely.

Ken twice participated in a one-month in-patient treatment session at Alcohol Foundation Manitoba. He also attended many evenings at AA (Alcoholics Anonymous). Nothing reached him until he spent three months in an out-of-province treatment facility. To everybody's great joy, he found the necessary help and follow-up support, and his next two years were alcohol-free! It was a happy time for all of us so heavily and emotionally involved.

Our optimism was guarded, and, sure enough, without warning, Ken slid back into drinking. This time he retreated more and more into a solitary lifestyle, and we recognized that things might not get better. For a long time, Ken managed to keep his job at the *Crisis Rehabilitation Unit*, but eventually the institution chose not to risk Ken's making a medical mistake with their vulnerable clientele, and he was dismissed.

This disastrous event appeared to cause Ken to give up. Addiction had struck again, only this time with an unforgiving power. No work, no salary, no friends, no future – only booze filled his hours.

This period of despair was, in some ways, more pain-filled for us than the months after he died. A normally neat, clean man, his condo was messy, and his clothes were unkempt. When I looked into his refrigerator, it was mostly empty, and I imagined the smell of *dying* long after I left the condo he had once loved so much. Ken's visits with Evan became tumultuous encounters between a dysfunctional addict and a teenager too young to understand what was happening.

Rather than give Ken money for groceries, we took him shopping. This caused him deep shame, and he could scarcely bear to choose the food he needed for normal living. One day, I half-filled the shopping cart, but when we got back to his condo, he sat silent and still in the car, literally unable to help put the food into his house. His guilt was profound.

Ken's frequent self-denigrating comments made me afraid for his life. With ever-increasing desperation, Betty and I continued seeking for alternative ways to find Ken assistance, but found a dearth of help for someone in his sick and frightful situation.

Although it caused me much pain to see Ken when he was not sober, I impulsively drove to his condo one late evening, a time of day he was most likely to be inebriated. The door to his condo was unlocked so I knocked, and walked in. He was slouched on his couch, and tried to get up when he saw me. I said, "Take it easy. It's all right," and slid down beside him and put my arm around his shoulders.

There is a time when a six-foot-tall drunken man, the smell of alcohol, and a half-empty bottle of vodka on the coffee table are not as important as the fact that the man is your son. Gone was my repugnance, my usual urge to leave, and my sense of disgrace. Instead, I remembered what it was like to hold our little baby boy in my arms and sing him to sleep. Ken's shoulders shifted restlessly under my arm and, on impulse, I began to sing:

Lullaby, and goodnight, with roses bedight
My little boy sleeps, goodnight, good night.
Close your eyes, fall asleep, I love you, I love you.
Close your eyes, fall asleep, I love you, I love you.

His head slid towards my chest, and I began a second lullaby:

Lu-a-a-lu-a-l-aby, all things now sleep 'neath the sky...

His head slipped lower, and I sang on, glad that I remembered the words. When I was done, he muttered "German one," and so I sang in German:

God's love is boundless, and full of mercy,
God's love is boundless, so full and free.

By the time I finished all the verses, his head was in my lap. I stretched my neck to see his face, and found him fast asleep. I sat for a long while – just Ken, my tears and the silence. When I finally disengaged myself, I covered him with a blanket, screwed the vodka bottle shut and left him there, locking the door behind me.

At home I said, "Betty, I think I said goodbye to Ken tonight," and we held each other, and wept until we were too tired to cry anymore.

Events moved from awful to tragic. Over several years, the Winnipeg Police had on occasion called us late at night asking if they could release Ken from their custody into ours. Their last call came very early one morning of August 2016. Ken had fallen and struck his head, they said. Paramedics found him unconscious, lying on the ground near his condo. They restarted his heart, drove him to the hospital where life supports breathed for him, and beat his heart for him. The police needed us to come identify him.

At the hospital, I reached over to comfort Betty who was touching Ken's face, holding his hands, trying to grasp what we could not wholly comprehend. His chest rose and fell with movements too precise to be his own. On the monitor, his heart appeared to be functioning normally, but we knew the hospital mechanisms were beating it for him. Nurses buzzed around the technical equipment, taking notes.

Soon Evan and Elaine arrived, and we watched as they absorbed this awful reality. Evan sat silently near his dad, oblivious of the nurses' commotion around him. Elaine, speechless and trembling, stared first at Ken and then at Evan, then back to Ken. Each of the four of us knew what was happening, but we needed time to absorb the harsh reality of the movie-like hospital scene, with Ken, unmoving, at its centre.

Jacquie was on a Quebec hiking trail, but we were happy her husband David joined our family catastrophe. Hospital staff tried to keep us up to date on what was actually an unchanging situation. Almost a week of this intensity continued, until a doctor suggested we all get together and decide what to do next. I nodded stiffly, stared at Ken and kissed his warm cheek. Betty and I stayed near each other, exchanging glances. Her hand was as cold as Ken's was warm.

The doctor reviewed the situation with us so we could come to a decision. To assist his brain in its possible recovery, Ken had been kept in a medically induced coma. For five days we had watched him lie immobile and totally unresponsive. His vitals could not manage on their own and, even if they met the five percent chance of recovery, his brain had been so seriously injured by the fall that, should he recover consciousness, his would be a life without meaning or understanding. None of us had ever made such a choice before, but we were unanimous in agreeing that the life supports should be withdrawn.

"All right," said the doctor, "Let's do it."

"Now?" we asked, almost simultaneously.

"Why should we wait?" asked the doctor, and we nodded at the common sense.

We took turns saying our last good-byes to Ken, except for Elaine and Evan, who chose to stay. The life supports were turned off, and we left, knowing that Kenneth James Neufeld, our Kenny, was effectually gone.

The day after saying our final farewell to Ken was a smear of sorrow on the pages of our lives. Lying on the dining room table, the funeral plans looked neat and tidy, but our minds felt smudged by an unwillingness to believe what was factual. The intellectual part of our brains planned efficiently, but emotionally the coming week looked like an unfocused movie on a wobbly screen.

We reached Jacquie again and let her know Ken had died. She was anxious to get home quickly, but we said we were coping not too badly, and suggested she not rush but come in ample time for the funeral, and plan to say something there. She agreed, and later told us the two friends she was travelling with were "like angels" in supporting her.

At home, Betty complained of a foggy mind. "Me, too," I said. "It's as though my five senses are hemmed in by a cloud." We picked up our pencils and kept sorting out the next week's sequence of events. Betty called our friend Dianne Cooper and asked if she felt steady enough to officiate at Ken's funeral. She said yes. Even though Ken had been her life-long friend, we knew she would get her tears under control by funeral time and contain them until later.

We asked Dianne to be open and honest with reference to Ken's alcohol addiction, and not to dodge that reality. A resolute woman of remarkable integrity, she readily agreed. Relieved, Betty and I continued organizing the many details which a funeral entails, even though we would much rather go cry somewhere, together.

How strange it felt to be at Ken's funeral. Evan's dad, so dear to his son, had taken his leave. The man whom Elaine loved for many years was dead. Our only son was ashes. Years of fearful anticipation had not prepared us for this confusion: loss, guilt, incomprehension, emptiness – and relief.

At the funeral, Dianne spoke in such a way as to reassure everyone, even while leaving a challenge. She had known Ken all his life, and let everyone know how much he was loved.

Dianne spoke candidly about his addiction, about how, for years, his family had tried to get assistance, and just how the dreadful illness afflicted Ken. Even though he was responsible for his actions, it seemed she saw him as a victim, and his final end a consequence of how society viewed addiction. I had never heard anyone speak so bluntly at a funeral about the overwhelming power of addiction, and how our society errs by ascribing full blame to the dead. Dianne's candid words comforted me, caused some mourners to breathe deeply – holding back tears – and others to study the floorboards. Those who loved Ken wept, and the full church united in silent mourning.

Years later, people still talk to me about the honest tone of the funeral, and its integrity. Despite the pain in Ken's life, Dianne reminded us how he also generated happiness and laughter with his family and his friends. Dianne's words demonstrated how Truth, even in the midst of acute pain, can begin to set us free.

After the funeral ceremonies were over, and a few hundred people gathered around informally, hugs and kisses touched us where words could not. What amazingly decent people my friends and relatives were, I thought. I had never felt such empathy in my lifetime, particularly now, when it was most needed.

At home, after the funeral, I moved restlessly from chair to chair, and found nothing I wanted to do. Staring at the wall, I tried to find some meaning in Ken's death – and could not. An emptiness as bare as Ken's condo enveloped me. I thought of the permanence of his absence, I imagined eternity, the never-ending-time it spawned, and wondered if I would ever experience Ken again.

When my parents died, I had moved through the anticipated grief, got through it, resumed normality – but I would never "get over" Ken's dying. I would feel no closure, as though something sad were over and we could go on with the rest of our lives. For Betty and me, it would *never* be over. She and I were both different people now, forever suffering a disseverance, a lasting sense of something having been sheared off, dismembered. We were two people who had once had a son.

Later that night, a silence spread like a bed cover over our condo. It reminded me how, as a boy, on a hot summer night, I used a big blanket to cover myself from forehead to toes when hiding from an approaching storm.

Evan

Evan's joyous birth occurred a few months after I retired, November 25, 1995. When we arrived at the hospital, Betty and I found the newborn Evan and his mother. I said to Betty, "He looks like me."

"No way. He's beautiful!" she said. We laughed, all of us on the edge of giddiness.

I said to Elaine, "How was it?"

She tried to smile but said, "I went through hell." I grimaced and shook my head, as if I could understand.

I had always wanted to add my own touch to this singular event. To be a different kind of grandpa had long been my desire, so, while Elaine was preoccupied with Betty and other visitors, I arranged our first grandson's tiny fingers in such a way that his middle finger pointed straight up to the ceiling while his other fingers lay bent back in his palm. The digits remained in place, and I skipped out of the hospital room.

A great cry of female indignation rang out, "Who did that! Oh, WHERE IS HANK?"

Ken had joined me in the hall, and by the time the women found us, their wrath had turned to reluctant grins. In his room with Elaine, the baby started to cry, and that gave me enough time to escape to the waiting room.

Later, Ken told me the baby's fingers had retained their layout, even though the women took turns trying to flatten them into what they called a *decent* position.

As planned, Elaine went back to work after arranging a good situation for Evan's care. Daily separation from their baby was a difficult adjustment for both parents, but it was a positive event for us because our baby grandchild stayed with us, beginning the first day away from home. Since Evan's birth coincided with my retirement, whenever Ken's and Elaine's work shifts overlapped, Betty or I picked up Evan and took him to our house. We sometimes kept him overnight, and, over time, developed a wonderful and intimate relationship. Betty, deeply delighted, often whispered to the baby that we were happy "to the moon and back."

As Evan grew, he learned to love water, whether it was the pool in a motel a few kilometres east on No. 1 Highway, or the huge pool in Winnipeg. He easily learned to swim, with enough confidence to, at least somewhat, reassure us about his safety.

Between our house and The Mint, the edge of a little lake captured his interest, and, as he got older, he caught water beetles and frogs. "Watch it paddle!" he exclaimed about a particularly big frog. "How can I make my legs longer so I can swim faster?" Betty always wished he could visit an uncle's farm to enhance his interest in the outdoors.

Evan must have spent time in school dreaming of "what would fit with what." He was fascinated with *Lego*, and became amazingly adept. On our way home from school one day, I bought him a miniature Lego airplane to assemble, and he had it put together before reaching the house. Hours flew by as he honed his aptitude and, like a pint-sized engineer, he taught himself building skills.

In his mid-teens, he turned his interest to cars. The Nissan Altima preoccupied him, and when Evan turned sixteen, he began planning how to own one. He easily passed a driver's test and began to drive his parents' Camry, and to save money. Grandma and Grandpa forked over some cash, he borrowed some money from nervous parents, he added his own savings and, at eighteen, he bought precisely the second-hand Nissan Altima which, over the years of saving, had gone down in price enough so he could afford it.

After graduating from Westgate Collegiate, he spent one unsatisfying month at the University of Manitoba. He dropped out, took a casual job and continued living alternatively between both his homes. He was exposed to his father's deteriorating lifestyle, which made for some miserable conflict. They had an early history of expressing their continuing love for each other, but this proved hard to do when the adult in the relationship consumed far too much vodka between work shifts.

Evan, sensitive as a gentle rainfall, was easily misdirected, and began having the occasional drink as well. He had half a dozen loyal friends his age who were stable young men and didn't let the odd party interfere with their lives. Evan, so distraught about his dad's drinking, and more susceptible than his friends, drank more often.

He was remarkably verbal with Betty and me about an overriding concern: If my dad loves me, why won't he stop drinking? Because of Betty's and my extensive reading, and through the sessions we attended in order to learn more about addiction, we came to accept a view which we applied to Evan, as we had to Ken: alcoholism was a disease, we told Evan, an addiction wielding a power so overwhelming, it caused alcoholics to sometimes treat those they loved very badly. I repeatedly told Evan that the most knowledgeable medical practitioners, usually doctors, viewed alcohol addiction as an illness. Blaming someone addicted to alcohol for his excessive drinking helped nothing. It was similar to blaming a man for having cancer. The only real help was intensive (group) treatment where addicts learned to know their *selves* better, where they dealt with personal issues that helped create the addiction, and they often learned life-saving ways to stay away from their addictive product. Surviving alcoholism took continuing hard work and an enormous commitment to become healthy. As well, we added, an addict's job was often at risk, and his dad was in danger of losing his employment. Finally, we talked about how hard it was to maintain decent relationships, and the ultimate outcome too often was death. Few alcoholics grew old.

When his dad died at age fifty-five, it was too much for Evan, and he fell into a depression from which he never recovered. Frightfully hurt, deeply offended and newly afraid that his mother, ill with a nasty prognosis, would also die, he got out of bed only for absolute necessities, like vodka.

A sudden heir to his father's various traits – and his estate – Evan followed Ken's path and almost immediately drank heavily, and quickly got caught up in addiction's web of "Gotcha!"

We spent as much time with Evan as he was able, and whenever he came to our house during a "dry" interval, he and Betty and I smothered him with affection and profound concern.

Over three months, Evan pulled himself together enough that he attended several alcohol-related day therapy sessions, and we helped him eventually schedule a long-term stay at an out-of-province addictions treatment. But his problems and his addiction were so overwhelming that one night, a series of drinking-related accidents led to his sudden death.

Hospital, Funeral and then Gone

I had often felt Evan was about to die, even though he had periods of sobriety when he would phone and say with youthful pride, "I've been sober for eight days." Then, in spite of great personal effort, he'd toboggan down addiction's steep hill where the rocks hid under the snow.

In July of 2019, his addiction proved stronger than life. Excessive drinking, a fall from his mom's outside deck, and a subsequent *grand mal* seizure forced a rush to the hospital. When we saw him, he was lying immobile in a room that dwarfed him. Stunningly like his father in physical appearance, identical tubes taped to his body led to the places designated to keep our so-young son and grandson in an induced coma.

Elaine sat beside his bed, holding Evan's still hand. Her pretty face showed the signs which extreme despair uncovers. The dreadful stress, too much for her beleaguered life, could not be hidden. Her sisters hovered nearby, trying to help, but addiction had claimed the family's second victim.

Evan was already beyond reach when a half dozen of his friends trooped in to say and sing goodbye, to kiss their buddy's forehead, and to cry. In their early twenties, they stood as witnesses to the innocence of youth gone awry. It must have been shocking for them to envision the alteration of Evan's normally handsome features, and to feel the imposition of death. They watched as a hospital machine indicated the descent of Evan's blood pressure until, along with his heart, it came to a full stop, and gentle Evan was gone.

If a much older person had lain in the coffin, perhaps the church attendees might have made some sense of the event, but a stone-dead twenty-three-year-old, a young man known for his gentleness and easy generosity, was dreadfully at odds with the verve and vitality of youth. People who had attended Ken's funeral a few years before must have been overcome by the sounds of the same people crying.

A week before his hospitalization, Evan and I had a conversation on the phone. The last thing he said was, "And give my special love to Grandma." He repeated, "Special, OK?"

I said, "For sure. Bye, Evan." I hung up the phone, and delivered the message.

Conclusion

Dr. Adam Menzies' forecast that I would be "a little Mennonite devil" proved at least half accurate. Mennonitism became an integral part of my being. I was born into the Anabaptist religion, and grew up under its imposing influence, so the Mennonite church's ethic remains as close as any I adhere to. I have questioned it, but I remain a Mennonite. Even while I seriously question its dogma, the

Mennonite church's ethic still dominates my sense of good and bad, right and wrong.

My church's interpretation of the Bible interfered with and complicated my thinking, but the underlying premise that God is the perpetual lover keeps circling my spiritual beliefs. This is true even though it seems most Mennonite churches' policy of excluding rather than including potential members conflicts with the Bible's insistence that God's unconditional love includes every human being regardless of behaviour or belief.

When I was nearing the age of eighty, the catastrophic deaths of two of my most-loved humans, my son and my grandson, threw a heavy wrench into my belief system. Their preventable double loss shook me like an angry cougar might shake a mouse. As though in a tornado, my personal resources twisted unreliably round and round. I viewed both deaths as lacking purpose and meaning. I still have not been able to reconcile the God of unconditional love with the omniscient God who could have salvaged both sick men – but didn't. I remain ignorant of solving this conundrum. The fact that Betty's indispensable love remains strong, and that the emotional support from a few dozen friends stays fast makes a huge difference. Ken's open smile, however, and the feel of Evan's arm around my shoulders haven't left me.

I don't understand where God fits into life's dreadful temporality. If I will see them again in a few years, why is this grief so acute, as though they are gone forever? I feel like the Old Testament's grieving father, David, who cried, "O Absalom, my son, my son. Would I had died for you. O Absalom, my son, my son!"

Two of my siblings are gone, and the other five wait for their timely turn. Although my earliest connection with my family members will always remain solidly fixed in my brain, their eventual dying will be appropriate, as a faded flower dying overnight. Not true for the death of "my two guys." What remains with no discernable meaning is their having been ripped out of our lives like a blown tire destroying a high-speed race car on a muddy track.

As the various clocks in Betty's and my condo keep ticking, the twin tragedies have become only slightly more believable. I am reminded, instead, of the more natural sense of life's end which followed my mother's death. I remember, too, how I gave a comfortable "yes" when my oldest sister, Kay, died. Or even when Papa died. Their deaths felt sadly right.

No such feelings came to me after Ken and Evan died. I pictured them in my mind constantly, and I cried bitterly; the peace I longed for kept its distance, and I talked nonstop about "my two guys" each chance I had.

Even misery, however, has its limits and before I could become a one-topic old man, Betty shared her own suffering with such remarkable openness and similitude that hopefulness edged my way. Nevertheless, I was forever changed, and will view the rest of my life through damaged eyes. It will feel like a miracle if I ever stop thinking about Ken and Evan each time I see a younger man throw his arms around his father or grandfather in simple, unadorned affection.

An Acknowledgement

Erica Ens proficiently edited this memoir even while assuming other roles. From previous experience, Erica's knowledge of book publishing proved essential. Her expertise with the computer was indispensable. She regularly presented creative suggestions for shaping this memoir, over a long period of time. Erica's steady assistance moved far beyond the second mile. She owns a deep integrity that is reflected in her work.

Erica translates diaries and letters from High German to English, including texts handwritten in Gothic script. She has also edited stories written in Low German.

CPSIA information can be obtained
at www.ICGtesting.com
Printed in the USA
BVHW081426060122
625106BV00002B/3